F. P. Chino   - CCHC

THE IUD

The IUD

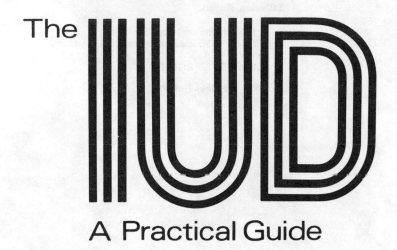

A Practical Guide

ROBERT SNOWDON, MARGARET WILLIAMS,
DENIS HAWKINS

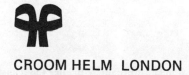

CROOM HELM LONDON

© 1977 Robert Snowdon, Margaret Williams, Denis Hawkins
Croom Helm Ltd, 2-10 St John's Road, London SW11

British Library Cataloguing in Publication Data

Snowdon, Robert
  The IUD.
  1. Intrauterine contraceptive.
  I. Title   II. Williams, Margaret   III. Hawkins,
  Denis
  613.9'435   RG137.3

  ISBN   0−85664−439−0

Printed in Great Britain by Biddles Ltd, Guildford, Surrey

CONTENTS

FOREWORD

This manual is intended to be a practical guide for those concerned with the fitting of intrauterine devices (IUDs) and with the subsequent care of those wearing an IUD. By linking the collective experience and treatment of the 20,000 IUD users described in this manual, we hope that those providing an IUD service will receive information of immediate and practical use.

We would like to express our thanks to the large number of people who have assisted the Family Planning Research Unit in its IUD research activities. Prominent among these is Dr Margaret Jackson whose early involvement in research into the use of IUDs led directly to the development of the Unit. The Family Planning Research Unit would not be able to operate without the collaboration of a large number of doctors, nurses and layworkers in the clinics taking part in the research network. Their work is recognised and appreciated and our thanks are extended to them all.

We would also like to thank the Pathfinder Fund for providing generous financial support during the early phases; the Family Planning Association for providing administrative assistance and the Medical Research Council for their help in setting up the project to provide national baselines for IUD use and effectiveness.

March 1977   R.S., M.W., D.H.

Clinics participating in the United Kingdom IUD Research Network are situated in:

Barnsley, Birmingham, Bridgwater, Bristol, Carlisle, Dorchester, Exeter, Glasgow, Guildford, London (2 centres), Norwich, Newport, Nuneaton, Plymouth, Sheffield, Southampton, Taunton and Woking.

SECTION I

THE INTRAUTERINE DEVICE

During the last forty years the climate of opinion regarding the IUD has shifted from one of outright condemnation to one of relative acceptance. A number of new IUD models have been designed and tested in the last decade and work on the development of new IUDs continues to the present time. The acceptance of the IUD as a method of contraception is not complete and arguments for and against its use are still widely debated. One of the principal reasons why the IUD has not achieved unqualified acceptance even with the present demand for methods of birth control is the lack of knowledge and guidance for those inserting the devices concerning the selection of the most appropriate device for the individual patient. It is a primary purpose of this manual to summarise knowledge and observed data in such a way as to provide that guidance.

Mode of Action

To date, it has not been possible to determine precisely at what point in the reproductive cycle the anti-fertility effect of the IUD is taking place. It is generally accepted that the principal contraceptive effect probably takes place within the uterus by interfering with the complex chain of events as the blastocyst becomes embedded in the endometrium. It is known that there are cellular changes in the endometrium in the presence of an IUD. The principal mode of action of the device is a creation of a hostile uterine environment through the effect of the IUD on the endometrial surface. It is also possible that the spermatozoa — and probably the blastocyst — which are in a vulnerable state whilst in the uterus, are directly affected by the uterine response to the presence of a foreign body.

The relationship between irritation and inflammation of the endometrial surface and prevention of nidation is complex and research continues to determine the precise mechanisms involved.

Theoretical and Use-Effectiveness of IUDs

Laboratory investigations of particular methods of birth control have placed much stress on those factors directly attributable to the intrinsic characteristics of the method. Consideration of the variation in the failure rates associated with a single birth control method among human populations has led researchers to differentiate between the 'theoretical effectiveness' of the method and its 'use-effectiveness'. The term 'theoretical effectiveness' is used to describe the use of the contraceptive under ideal conditions, where it is used consistently and exactly according to instructions. This level of effectiveness can only remain as a theoretical concept for such conditions hardly exist. 'Use-effectiveness' refers to the level of contraceptive efficiency achieved by an individual or couple under the conditions of everyday life. Use-effectiveness of a method therefore incorporates its theoretical or laboratory effectiveness but also includes the human factor involved in the provision and use of the method.

The United Kingdom IUD Research Programme

Research into the provision and use of IUDs has been taking place at the University of Exeter since 1968. The Family Planning Research Unit was formally established within the Department of Sociology on 1 July 1971.

The Unit is primarily concerned with the evaluation of the factors that may be present in IUD acceptance and in subsequent continuation or rejection of the IUD as a contraceptive method. To undertake research of this kind the Unit administers a data retrieval system designed to facilitate the systematic collection of information pertaining to the use of IUDs being fitted in twenty centres in the United Kingdom. These centres provide information on about 6,000 new IUD acceptors each year with follow-up information on these women for as long as they continue to use this method of contraception. The feedback of information from this nationally coordinated network of research clinics provides basic data on IUD effectiveness and complications. In addition to the study of the medical factors in IUD use-effectiveness, the Unit examines social and personal factors relating to the IUD acceptor, the person fitting the IUD, and the institution providing the IUD service.

This manual is based on the information supplied by these twenty centres between April 1972 and July 1976, relating to just over 20,000 IUD fittings.

LEVELS OF IUD ASSESSMENT

The evaluation of IUDs provided for use as part of a family planning service is usually undertaken at one or more of three conceptually distinct but overlapping levels. These are: (1) preliminary assessment; (2) limited clinical trials; (3) general clinical trials.

When a device is received for clinical assessment the first step is to decide at which level such assessment is to be undertaken. The level at which an assessment is made depends on the quantity and quality of the background information already available in relation to a specific device. This decision will, to a large extent, determine the procedures to be followed.

Preliminary Assessment

The most obvious example of assessment at this level relates to the entirely new IUD which is being seriously considered for limited clinical testing for the first time. Before such clinical trials are commenced, it is customary to obtain the views of clinicians, gynaecologists and researchers concerning the suitability of the device for a trial. A similar assessment is often made when an IUD is being introduced into this country for the first time irrespective of the availability of background information obtained elsewhere.

The preliminary assessment report consists of a collated account of the comments expressed by the medical consultants. This provides a basis for deciding whether or not the IUD concerned should be tested in a limited clinical trial. As a result of the views expressed, some IUDs are withdrawn, some modified and others forwarded to the appropriate official body to whom a request for a clinical trial certificate is made.

Limited Clinical Trial

In a limited clinical trial a single clinic or a small number of clinics are provided with a number of devices to be fitted in a group of women. Progress with the device, including the occurrence of side effects, is carefully monitored by means of a rigorous follow-up procedure. The limited clinical trial is concerned principally with an assessment of the medical safety of the device and its effectiveness in preventing pregnancy. Because the trial is necessarily carried out under controlled conditions requiring a pre-selected group of acceptors, data obtained does not necessarily give a valid indication of the acceptability of the device among the general population of potential IUD users.

General Clinical Trial

A general clinical trial is intended to approximate more closely to actual situations in the general provision of IUDs. Data is collected from several medical teams fitting substantial numbers of IUDs in clinics situated in a variety of geographical locations in England, Scotland and Wales. Assessment at this level is concerned not only with an evaluation of medical factors but also with personal and social factors which may affect the acceptability and effectiveness of IUDs in general and specific IUD models in particular.

Analysis Procedures

The common method in measuring the failure or success of any contra-ceptive method before 1930 was by reference to the proportion of unplanned pregnancies to the total number of users of the method of contraception under discussion. This method took no account of the period of exposure to possible pregnancy and for this reason was far from accurate in estimating failure rates. In 1932 Pearl published a formula which took into account this period of exposure to risk of pregnancy. His 'rate per 100 woman years' (HWY) or 'Pearl Index' (Appendix) is still extensively used. The development of the life-table approach in the 1960s was considered an important advance in the prediction of risks associated with different contraceptive methods. Life-table analysis takes into account not only the total period of risk using a specific birth control method but also any shift in the monthly probability of such risk. In short this approach gives the probability of a defined risk occurring by the Nth month following fitting of an IUD. An advantage with the life-table method is the ability to assess defined risks in the presence of other competing risks. With the IUD the risk of pregnancy must be seen in relation to the risk of expulsion and removal of the device if the overall use and effectiveness of the device is to be ascertained. The results are presented as 'use-effectiveness' rates.

THE IUD USER

The suitability of an IUD for use as a contraceptive is related to the age and parity of the woman concerned. Other considerations include the degree of certainty with which a pregnancy should be avoided, the medical history and the current medical health of the candidate.

Age and Parity

The tables given in Section II of this manual provide information on a number of categories relating to age and parity as independent of each other and also as interacting variables. The most useful classification has been found to be:

1. Parity

    a) Nulliparous
    b) Low parity — one or two previous pregnancies
    c) High parity — three or more previous pregnancies

2. Age

    a) Low age (under thirty years)
    b) High age (thirty years or over)

Reproductive Future

No method of contraception is 100 per cent effective in preventing pregnancy, and the acceptability of different levels of risk is also important. This acceptability is clearly related to whether or not a future pregnancy is desired. There are three categories regarding future pregnancy: (1) the delayer — the patient who is delaying her first pregnancy; (2) the spacer — the patient who has experienced at least one pregnancy and is anticipating another sometime in the foreseeable future; (3) the stopper — the patient who definitely does not wish to have a pregnancy in the future. Although the delayer is nulliparous, some nulliparous women are also 'stoppers' in that no future pregnancy is desired. Parous women are either 'spacers' or 'stoppers' depending on their desire for a future pregnancy.

These categories of potential IUD candidates introduce an element of motivation into the use of the IUD and this will interact in varying degrees with the age and parity categories. For example, a patient who is under thirty years of age, who has a parity of one or two and who definitely does not want another pregnancy is very different from a woman of similar age and parity but who is spacing pregnancies. These differences are important in relation not only to patient acceptability of the chance of an unwanted pregnancy but also to the toleration of side effects associated with IUD use.

Description of IUD Candidate

The following account of patient characteristics is intended as a guide for those contemplating the fitting of an IUD. In describing the IUD candidate the experience of the IUD users providing data in the United Kingdom is supplemented by the reported experience of doctors responsible for the fitting of IUDs.

Whether or not an IUD fitting should be undertaken is related to the reported experience of these women wearing IUDs but note should also be made of the alternative methods available at any given time. The medical, social and psychological risks associated with an unplanned and unwanted pregnancy often outweigh those of wearing an IUD, even amongst those for whom the IUD is not considered to be the wisest choice. Higher risks may well be associated with alternative methods of contraception. Care should be taken that advice is not given which causes the patient to be placed at more risk than she is facing with her previous contraceptive method.

The Nulliparous Patient

Even with devices fitted by means of a small diameter inserter such as the Gravigard (Copper 7) the discomfort at fitting is undoubtedly greater for the nulliparous woman than for one who has borne children in recent years. This is not to suggest that the nulliparous patient should never be fitted with an IUD — circumstances should determine this. Before undertaking such a fitting, the possible attendant

14

difficulties should be discussed.

The United Kingdom data suggest that the IUD should not be the first choice of fertility regulation for nulliparous patients and serious consideration should be given to alternative methods of contraception. Despite the recent introduction of IUDs for this category of patient the following points should be considered:

1. Insertion is generally more difficult.
2. The pregnancy risk is somewhat higher than with oral contraceptives.
3. There is an increased risk of pelvic inflammatory disease among IUD users and a link is claimed with subsequent infertility.
4. If this category of patient is discouraged from using the IUD owing to an unwanted pregnancy or unacceptable side effects, the experience may militate against the use of an IUD even when her subsequent age, parity and reproductive status would make the method highly desirable.

These problems are accentuated in nulliparae irrespective of age (see Section II).

Nulliparous Patient: No Future Pregnancy Desired

The general difficulties associated with IUD use by nulliparous patients are increased in this group where a pregnancy is definitely not desired in the foreseeable future. These patients — often single girls — need to use a method which is particularly effective in preventing pregnancy. It must also be remembered that an IUD will not provide protection against venereal disease and the risk of pelvic inflammatory disease.

Nulliparous Patient: Delaying First Pregnancy

The most serious question in this situation is the small possibility of pelvic inflammatory disease and the effect of this on subsequent fertility. There is a small risk of pregnancy but an unplanned pregnancy arriving earlier than expected need not be such a problem for this patient. A small proportion of patients with unproven fertility are, in any case, subfertile. All nulliparous women should be warned of this possibility for, if they are unable to conceive after wearing an IUD, they may erroneously blame the IUD for the subfertility.

The Parous Patient

Women who have had children are good candidates for IUD use. There is a small chance of a pregnancy after an IUD has been fitted but this tends to decrease with increasing age of the patient as her fecundity diminishes. Section II provides details of the most common events associated with specific IUDs for women in different age and parity groups.

Low Parity (1 and 2) Patient: Spacing Pregnancies	The ideal IUD candidate. The small risk of pregnancy is not such a problem with this patient.
Low Parity (1 and 2) Patient: No Further Pregnancy Desired	The risk of pregnancy makes this patient not quite as suitable as the parous patient who is currently spacing pregnancies. Age plays an important part in relation to the level of risk. By and large, the older woman has a lower level of fecundity than the younger woman but serious consideration should be given to more permanent methods of contraception if this patient is certain that she desires no further pregnancy.
High Parity (3 and over) Patient: Spacing Pregnancies	Also an ideal IUD candidate. A small risk of pregnancy still remains but evidence suggests that with most devices the expulsion rate is lower and the incidence of bleeding and pelvic pain are reduced compared with patients in lower parity groups.
High Parity (3 and over) Patient: No Further Pregnancy Desired	Notice that there is still some risk of pregnancy. An unplanned pregnancy may be particularly inconvenient for this type of patient and more permanent methods of contraception should be considered. If sterilisation is not acceptable and an IUD is the method chosen then an adjunctive method of contraception should be used as well if the patient desires maximum protection.
The Post-partum Patient	About seven weeks post-partum is generally considered to be a good time for fitting an IUD. The post-partum patient who is spacing pregnancies is an ideal IUD candidate. If no further pregnancies are desired an alternative method should be considered because of the small chance of pregnancy with an IUD. Immediate post-partum fittings are carried out in some hospitals but this approach is not part of a routine IUD service.
The Post-abortum Patient	Immediate post-abortum IUD fittings have been carried out but these have generally been undertaken as part of carefully planned clinical trials. In the more general situation the same considerations as for post-partum fittings apply.
The Menopausal Patient	Patients approaching the menopause are relatively good candidates for IUD use since the natural cessation of menstruation is not masked as it may be if oral contraceptives are being used. Once a woman has

passed the menopause an IUD should not be left *in situ*. As renewal of the endometrial surface is no longer taking place, the uterine wall gradually becomes atrophic, and perhaps less resistant to erosion by the device.

Unstable Marital or Sexual Relationship

Before fitting an IUD the problems of difficulty of follow-up, lack of protection against venereal disease and risk of pregnancy should be considered. The situation of 'any method better than none' and the social and medical risks associated with an unplanned and unwanted pregnancy (should either no method or a less effective alternative method be used) also deserve careful consideration.

Psychiatric Illness

Consultation with the specialist concerned should be sought before fitting an IUD. The risk of expulsion and possible pregnancy should be weighed against the advantages associated with IUD use. Unlike most other methods of contraception, the IUD may not require sustained motivation in its use, but it does require sustained motivation to ensure that it has not been expelled.

Previous IUD Expulsion

Most IUD fitting doctors try to persevere with 'chronic' IUD expellers by refitting a different IUD model; especially one which, by its design, is known to be difficult to expel. The generally available IUD which is often used for this purpose is the Antigon device. Many doctors find this device difficult to fit. Refitting a larger size of the same IUD model is unlikely to reduce the risk of expulsion and, in addition, complaints concerning an increase in bleeding and pain are often made. Alternative methods of contraception should seriously be considered.

THE PATIENT'S MEDICAL HISTORY

Difficult Pregnancy or Confinement	There is no reported effect of a previous difficult pregnancy or confinement on subsequent IUD fitting and use. Trauma sustained by the uterus and cervix at delivery may later effect the successful use of an IUD. It should be borne in mind that an IUD may be the only acceptable method for women for whom oestrogen-containing contraceptives are contra-indicated (e.g. recent thrombosis or hepatitis, jaundice during pregnancy, etc.).
Caesarean Section	In theory, there is a possibility of perforation through the uterine scar if an IUD is fitted. This has not been substantiated in practice. If in doubt the patient should be referred to a gynaecologist for fitting.
Suspicion of Pregnancy	If there is a possibility that conception may have occurred since the last menstrual period it is unwise to fit an IUD until pregnancy has been excluded.
Recent Irregular Bleeding	An IUD should not be fitted. The cause of irregular bleeding should be determined and, where appropriate, treated before a fitting is undertaken.
Menorrhagia	It is unwise to fit an IUD in a patient with undiagnosed menorrhagia; the condition should be investigated and treated. An IUD is not a first choice of contraceptive method for a patient with menorrhagia which is known to be functional in origin; it may exacerbate the symptoms. If no other method is acceptable then close medical supervision should be maintained.
Pelvic Inflammatory Disease (PID)	Diagnosis of PID may be difficult and a reported history of this condition is often hard to evaluate. Many doctors consider a past history of PID to be a contra-indication to IUD use, even when the patient has been free of trouble for months or years. If an IUD is fitted, a watch should be kept for possible recurrence of PID. It is known that IUD users experience PID at a higher rate than non-users and those already having a history of PID are at particular risk.
Fibroids	The IUD is inappropriate for patients with large or multiple fibroids, owing to a relatively high risk of perforation at insertion, pregnancy, expulsion and menorrhagia.

Dysplasia or Carcinoma in situ of the Cervix	There is no evidence of a relationship between IUD use and cancer, nor is there evidence which associates IUD use with the transition from cervical dysplasia to carcinoma *in situ* or to invasive cancer. A patient who has been treated by cone biopsy can be successfully fitted with an IUD. If in doubt consultation with the gynaecologist who carried out the cone biopsy is indicated.
Previous Operations on the Uterus	Previous operations on the fundus of the uterus may predispose to perforation of the uterus. Previous operations on the cervix may cause scar tissue, rendering insertion difficult. If in doubt, the patient should be referred to a specialist for IUD fitting.
Previous Perforation of Uterus	Try to find out why this happened. An IUD may subsequently be safely fitted but if in doubt the patient should be referred to a gynaecologist.
Anaemia	Heavier menstrual blood loss is usual following an IUD fitting. The anaemia should be diagnosed and treated before an IUD is fitted.
Chest Disease	The IUD may introduce infection which can have serious consequences for these patients. Specialist advice should be sought before fitting an IUD.
Pulmonary Tuberculosis	An IUD can be considered for these patients if their disease is under treatment or quiescent.
Rheumatic Heart Disease; Congenital Heart Disease; Renal Disease	There is a chance that the IUD may introduce infection which, if it enters the blood stream, can have serious consequences for patients with a history of these diseases. Alternative methods of contraception should be considered.
Diabetes	Some doctors consider that an IUD carries fewer risks for the diabetic than the use of oral contraception.
Epilepsy	This should not affect IUD fitting and use. It is reported that an epileptic seizure can occur at or shortly after IUD fitting. The possibility that this may happen should be borne in mind.
Anticoagulant Drugs	The amount of bleeding following an IUD fitting in a woman on anticoagulants may be unacceptable. If no other form of contraception seems appropriate, the patient should be referred for a specialist opinion.

Steroid Therapy   An IUD may be fitted but the possible masking of pelvic inflammatory disease developing with IUD use should be considered.

IUD FITTING AND EXAMINATION

Introduction   When fitting an IUD, it is essential that the correct procedures are followed with gentleness and consideration for the patient concerned. Skill, speed and the ability to convey confidence contribute to successful IUD fitting and use.

Preliminary Discussion with Patient   A medical, obstetric and gynaecological history should be taken to rule out possible contra-indications to the method. The patient should be informed of the side effects which she may experience following fitting of the device. This should include a discussion of the risk of pregnancy. To help relieve anxiety the fitting procedure should be briefly explained.

**QUESTIONS OFTEN
ASKED BY PATIENTS**

1.   *Will the IUD cause cancer?*
There is good evidence that the use of an IUD does not predispose the wearer to either cervical or endometrial cancer.

2.   *What is the risk of unwanted pregnancy?*
On average there is a chance of about 3 in 100 that any one IUD user will become pregnant in any one year. There is some variation in this chance depending on the type of IUD being fitted and the age and parity of the woman concerned. The IUD is a little less efficient than the pill in preventing pregnancy.

3.   *For how long will the IUD be effective?*
Most IUDs can be left in the uterus for several years without harmful effect. Some devices should be replaced every two years (e.g. the Copper 7 or the Copper T) and some should be replaced at shorter intervals (e.g. the Progestasert).

4.   *Will I be able to have a baby after I have ceased using the IUD?*
It is estimated that one third of all women wishing to conceive after IUD removal do so within one month of removal. Almost 3 out of 4 do so within 6 months, and 9 out of 10 within one year. Future fertility rates are somewhat lower in women of unproved fertility, a proportion of whom are infertile, and in older women, particularly those over forty.

5.   *How soon can I have sex after IUD fitting?*
Protection against pregnancy is immediate.

6.   *Should I take any special precautions in the first few months?*
The incidence of displacement or expulsion is highest then; you should check the device is in place each week if you wish to be very careful.

7.   *How do I know the IUD is in place?*
You will be shown how to feel for the tail of the IUD. The tail consists of two threads which can be felt with the fingers once you know where to feel.

8.   *Will the IUD make my periods worse?*
The first two or three periods after the IUD is fitted may be heavier than usual but this will normally settle.

9.   *How often do I have to come for checks?*

Clinic or practice procedure should be explained.

10.   *Is the IUD difficult to remove?*
There is normally no difficulty in IUD removal.

11.   *If I do have a baby when wearing an IUD, will the baby be affected?*
Not all pregnancies succeed in going to term but those that do show that the IUD is not related to any abnormality in the baby. The chances of having a completely normal baby are as good for the mother wearing an IUD as for the mother who is not wearing an IUD.

Husband's Agreement to IUD Fitting

An indication should be made in the notes at the time of IUD fitting that the patient has agreed to the IUD procedure. A note should be made also of the patient's marital status and, where appropriate, that she has discussed the IUD fitting with her husband who also agrees to the IUD fitting. If in doubt use a consent form which the patient should sign. This form should include the words 'and my husband/partner also agrees'.

The insertion of an IUD is a minor surgical procedure with an attendant morbidity and mortality, however small. It is therefore unwise to fit an IUD to a girl under sixteen years of age without the knowledge and consent of a parent. It is unethical to fit an IUD to a mentally disturbed patient who is incapable of appreciating the nature and function of the device.

When to Fit an IUD

An IUD can be fitted at any time in the menstrual cycle but most doctors prefer to fit during menstruation or just after. This makes it unlikely that a pregnancy is present and the cervix is easier to negotiate at this time. There is the additional advantage that slight blood loss occurring as a result of the fitting procedure will not be so noticeable. Consideration should be given to the embarrassment some patients may experience if they are requested to attend for IUD fitting when they are actually menstruating.

Post-partum or Post-abortum Patients

Post-partum or post-abortum patients are not usually fitted with an IUD before six to eight weeks have elapsed since the delivery or abortion. Some fittings are done at delivery or termination of pregnancy or soon after but these are usually undertaken in hospital. Ease of fitting at this time is an advantage but devices fitted in the early post-partum or post-abortum period are associated with a higher risk of expulsion and perforation.

Uniformly good results have been reported with devices fitted six to eight weeks after delivery. This is a convenient time for the procedure; a six- to eight-week postnatal examination is commonly part of routine obstetric care.

There is some conflict of opinion concerning the fitting of an IUD immediately after treatment for an incomplete abortion. The abortion may be associated with pelvic infection and the fitting of an IUD might exacerbate this condition. There is also a small risk of perforation of the uterus.

What to Fit

This depends on the availability of the IUD model, the size and shape of the uterus, the age and parity of the patient and whether or not the patient is delaying her first pregnancy, is spacing pregnancies or intends to have no further pregnancy. An additional consideration may be the patient's previous experience with an IUD. Section II provides details of the advantages and disadvantages of specific IUD models in relation to most of these variables.

Note should be made not only of the size, shape and configuration of the IUD in relation to the patient but also of the size and malleaability of the device inserter. The size of the inserter varies according to the size and type of IUD being fitted. A comparison of inserter sizes is given in Section II in association with the description of specific IUD models. The smaller the outside diameter of the inserter the less likely it is that trauma will be inflicted on a small cervical canal and internal os. With larger inserters it may be necessary to dilate the cervix slightly (to 4, 5 or even 6 Hegar).

Routine replacement after an interval of one to two years is advised with some devices (e.g. Copper 7, Copper T, Progestasert) and the choice of these devices will be affected by the confidence in the patient's willingness (or ability) to return for follow-up.

In general, it is better to fit those IUDs of which the person responsible for the fitting has some experience. The data collected from a large number of centres and doctors indicate that there is a wider variation in successful IUD fitting and use between these doctors than there is between different IUD models or sizes. Skill and regular practice are needed if the confidence of patients — which is so necessary to the successful use of an IUD — is to be maintained.

THE FITTING EXAMINATION

The objectives of this examination are to ascertain the condition of vagina, cervix and cervical canal, and the position, size and condition of the uterus.

Position of Patient

Most doctors find that it is easier to fit an IUD with the patient in the dorsal or lithotomy position. The important criteria are comfort for the patient and good visibility for the person undertaking the IUD fitting. A suitable couch, with lithotomy poles attached, is a useful piece of equipment although not essential.

A few doctors prefer the left lateral position because they believe this causes less embarrassment to the patient, but this is not generally recommended.

Examination Procedures

With the patient in position the first step is to undertake a general examination of the vulva, vagina and cervix. A bivalve speculum is inserted into the vagina to permit visualisation of the vagina and cervix. If there is excessive or abnormal vaginal discharge present a diagnosis should be established and suitable treatment undertaken before an IUD is fitted. Consideration should be given to the alternative risks facing the patient presenting with an excessive or abnormal vaginal discharge in the event of a decision being made not to fit an IUD. In mild cases of trichomoniasis or candidiasis an IUD fitting is sometimes undertaken but most doctors prefer to clear up the infection first. If gonorrhoea is suspected the IUD should not be fitted before treatment has been completed.

The routine taking of Papanicolaou smears should be carried out when an IUD is fitted unless the patient has recently had a smear examined. The fitting of an IUD is a convenient time to perform preventive medical procedures such as a cervical smear. Apart from carcinoma *in situ*, unsuspected trichomonal, candidal or virus infections may be detected in a smear. It is preferable to take the smear before doing the bimanual examination (i.e. before placing a finger in the vagina).

Attention should be paid to the state of the cervical os and canal. The most difficult task in fitting an IUD is the negotiation of the cervix.

A bimanual examination of the uterus is then performed. Careful palpation of the cervix may add to the information on its state obtained by inspection. The position (anteverted, axial or retroverted) of the uterus, any extreme degree of uterine flexion, and uterine size, consistency and mobility are examined as well as noting any tenderness on movement and palpating any associated masses. The right and left adnexa are then felt bimanually in turn. Normal tubes and ovaries are often impalpable. If an ovary is felt an opinion as to its normality in size and consistency should be formed. The main purpose of examining the adnexa is to detect tenderness or thickening, which may indicate pelvic inflammatory disease, and to detect ovarian cysts or other pelvic tumours. Mild vague generalised tenderness of the pelvic organs can be associated with normal menstruation, but localised tenderness or significant discomfort on movement of the pelvic organs suggests abnormality.

Some doctors prefer to perform a bimanual examination before passing a speculum, as the instrument does not then have to be removed and later replaced for IUD insertion. Most doctors are trained to inspect before they palpate and perhaps disturb the findings.

Abnormalities Detected on Pelvic Examination

Cervical Erosion

A high proportion of post-partum women have some degree of cervical erosion and this can be ignored. If the erosion is large and florid some doctors prefer to treat the erosion and delay the IUD fitting. If the patient will return for a fitting on another occasion and is willing to take other precautions in the meantime, a delay in IUD fitting may be recommended until the erosion has healed. Otherwise, it is possible to cauterise the erosion or apply a cryoprobe and fit the IUD at once.

Lacerated Cervix; Patulous Cervix

If the internal os is competent an IUD can be fitted. If the internal os is damaged the risk of expulsion is high. If an IUD is fitted it is particularly important that the patient should check the presence of the IUD frequently by feeling for the tail. This should be done regularly, and certainly after each menstrual period.

Cervical Polyp

The patient should be referred for treatment before an IUD is fitted.

Acutely Anteflexed or Anteverted Uterus

If the uterus is acutely anteflexed it may be necessary to use traction on a tenaculum applied to the cervix to line up the axis of the cervical canal with that of the uterus. Particular care must be taken to avoid perforation if the uterus is sounded and during IUD fitting. If difficulty is encountered, the patient should be referred to a specialist for IUD fitting.

Retroverted Uterus

If the uterus is fixed in this position the patient should be referred to a gynaecologist for assessment and possible IUD fitting. If the uterus is mobile, there should be little difficulty in fitting an IUD if traction on the cervix is performed with a tenaculum. Particular care should be taken to avoid perforation when sounding the uterus or during insertion.

Bulky Uterus

Check carefully for possible pregnancy or fibroids. Do not fit an IUD until the reason for the enlargement has been ascertained.

Fibroids

Do not fit an IUD until this condition has been assessed by a gynaecologist. If the fibroids affect the shape of the uterine cavity this will affect the position of the IUD and may induce pain and bleeding. The risk of pregnancy will be increased.

Pelvic Inflammatory Disease

A history of vaginal discharge, pelvic pain and abnormal menstruation suggest this condition. Physical findings may include uterine tenderness, parametrial or adnexal tenderness, and adnexal thickening or masses. An IUD should not be fitted and reference to a gynaecologist is indicated.

Other Gynaecological Disorders

Ectopic gestation, ovarian cysts or endometriosis may rarely be encountered. If any of these conditions is suspected, the IUD should not be fitted and the patient should be referred to a gynaecologist.

FITTING THE IUD

Cleaning of Cervix

It is more important to clean vaginal secretions and debris from the cervix than to attempt to create a completely sterile condition. Sterile cotton wool swabs and an antiseptic solution such as benzalkonium chloride, cetrimide, chlorhexidine or hexachlorophane should be used.

Use of Tenaculum

A single toothed tenaculum or vulsellum is usually used to steady the uterus and to draw it into the axis of the cervical canal for greater ease of IUD fitting. The tenaculum does cause discomfort to the patient and there are differing views on its use. Some consider that a tenaculum should be used if more than a small degree of flexion of the uterus exists in relation to the axis of the cervical canal. The most helpful advice in relation to this issue is that the procedure with which the doctor has become familiar in training or through experience should be followed. When a tenaculum is used it is best used to grip the anterior or lateral vaginal aspect of the cervix.

Sounding of Uterus

Sounding of the uterus before IUD fitting is considered to be essential by most IUD fitting doctors, though a few feel equally strongly that it predisposes to perforation. Confirmation of the uterine size, shape and position can be obtained by the use of a sound. Again, the doctor should be guided by his training and experience.

As an additional precautionary measure against contamination and to permit easier access, some doctors apply a small amount of antiseptic cream to the tip of the sterile sound and inserter before they are introduced into the cervical canal.

The sound should pass through the cervical canal easily. If resistance is encountered care should be taken to ensure that perforation does not result. If difficulty is encountered in negotiating the cervical canal the patient is asked to return when she is menstruating or an antispasmodic such as amyl nitrite by inhalation is used. Additional care should be exercised if the uterus is believed to be acutely anteflexed or retroflexed.

In cases of uterine abnormality (e.g. if a uterine septum or bicornuat uterus are suspected) consultation with a specialist is indicated before an IUD is fitted.

Dilatation of Internal Os

This is sometimes necessary to permit the passage of the larger size IUD inserters and for women with a cervical canal that is difficult to negotiate. The passage of a Hegar 3 or 4 dilator is sufficient for insertion of the Lippes Loop but this will be insufficient for the fitting of larger devices such as the Antigon. It is better to dilate the cervix to Hegar 5 or 6 than to damage the wall of the cervical canal with an IUD inserter. Some doctors advocate the use of intracervical or paracervical blocks with a local anaesthetic to facilitate dilatation of the cervix. Most feel that the discomfort caused by insertion of the block is greater than that due to careful dilatation.

Loading IUD into Inserter

This should be undertaken using a 'no-touch' technique. The instructions provided with the IUD should be followed very closely. Ensure that the device is correctly placed in the inserter and that no part protrudes more than it should beyond the end of the inserter. The IUD should not normally be left in the inserter for more than a few minutes before fitting as this will affect the 'memory' of the device on its release in the uterus.

Fitting Procedure

It is believed that most perforations occur at the time of IUD fitting and therefore great care should be taken. The procedure varies according to the device and care should be taken to follow the instructions provided with the IUD. Most modern IUDs are supplied with a hollow inserter tube into which the IUD is loaded. Once the inserter and IUD are passed along the cervical canal and into the uterine cavity, the IUD is either pushed out of the inserter tube by means of a plunger inserted into the free end of the inserter or is left in the uterus by holding the plunger steady against the device and slowly withdrawing the inserter tube. These two procedures are in some ways opposite to each other and should confusion between them occur the danger of uterine perforation is increased.

A third group of IUDs have a carrying rod and are thrust through the cervix. The device is compressed by its passage through the cervical canal and re-expands inside the uterine cavity. IUDs requiring this type of insertion are, in general, unsuitable if the cervical canal is tight. The doctor should be confident of the position of the uterus and it is desirable that he should have been specially trained in the use of the device concerned.

Irrespective of the technique used, it is important that the IUD is released in the transverse plane of the uterus. Once in position, the fitting instruments should be removed slowly and carefully to minimise discomfort to the patient and avoid catching the tail of the IUD, which may dislodge the device.

The actual fitting procedure normally takes a minute or two and should proceed without difficulty in the majority of cases. Little or no force should be used to accomplish the IUD fitting. If undue resistance is encountered then the fitting should be abandoned and a decision made about another attempt after a re-evaluation of the situation. One common error is where an inserter designed to enter the uterine cavity remains in the cervical canal at the internal os. In such cases the end of the device may be left in the cervical canal after ejection from the inserter tube. This usually causes pain and subsequent expulsion of the device.

Anxious Patient with Tight Cervix

If the cervical canal is difficult to negotiate consider: (1) requesting the patient to return when she is menstruating — the cervix will be less tight at that time; (2) inhalation of amyl nitrite at the time of fitting to reduce spasm; (3) dilatation of the cervical canal by a small amount (Hegar 4). Do not proceed with IUD fitting if the patient cannot relax. There is then a higher risk of perforation.

Local anaesthesia with an intracervical or paracervical block is of little use in these patients. They are the group who are least able to relax to permit insertion of the block and who are the least tolerant of the discomfort involved.

Cervical Shock

Very rarely (approximately 1 in 1,000 fittings) a patient will collapse when a sound is passed through the cervix, when dilatation of the cervix is attempted or the inserter is introduced into the cervix. The common cause is vaso-vagal syncope, characterised by a high pulse, a rather low blood pressure and a cold and moist skin. If the patient's condition does not rapidly improve on resting in the supine position, atropine sulphate, 0.6 mg, should be given intravenously. A rare cause is an unsuspected cardiovascular condition such as paroxysal tachycardia or a Stokes-Adams attack. Another is unsuspected epilepsy and convulsive movements suggest the need for an intravenous anti-convulsant such as diazepam, 10 mg. With older women the small chance that a coronary thrombosis or a cerebral vascular accident has occurred should not be forgotten.

Even if the cause is believed to be simple syncope, the patient should be referred for a specialist medical opinion before any further attempt to fit a device is made.

Trimming of IUD Tail

Trim the tail of the IUD so that about 3 cm is left in the vagina. There are usually two strings to the tail.

ADVICE TO PATIENT AFTER FITTING

1. Instructions should be given for checking the presence of the IUD tail by digital palpation of the cervix and the suggestion made that this is done after each menstrual period.
2. The presence of the tail in the vagina should not affect sexual intercourse and the husband or partner will not normally feel it. If the partner does complain the patient should return.
3. The patient should be advised to return if the bleeding or pain experienced at fitting continues for more than a day or two or simple analgesics do not help. If she develops symptoms of pyrexia she should see a doctor at once.
4. The patient should be advised to return if she encounters any other difficulty which she associates with the IUD.
5. She should be informed that she should expect heavier blood loss during the next two or three periods but that this should settle down subsequently.
6. Some back ache may be experienced and, occasionally, pelvic or

abdominal pain. If there is significant discomfort the patient should return.

7. The small risk of pregnancy when using an IUD should be discussed, and where it is felt to be desirable, use of a suitable adjunctive method may be advised. Some doctors advise the use of spermicides or of barrier procedures at the mid-cycle, to achieve maximum protection against pregnancy.

8. The importance of follow-up visits should be emphasised, especially where the contraceptive life of the IUD is known to be limited. With inert devices patients appreciate the need for a 'check up' to verify that the device is properly in place and 'working satisfactorily'.

IMMEDIATE POST-FITTING COMPLICATIONS

Suspicion of Perforation at Fitting

A perforation should be suspected if:

1. the sound enters the uterus further than it should (e.g. 4 to 5 inches; 8 to 11 cm) and no resistance is felt;
2. the inserter enters the uterus further than it should;
3. the patient complains of sudden pelvic pain and abdominal tenderness (note that not all such cases indicate the occurrence of perforation)
4. after removal of inserter, the IUD tail cannot be seen in the vagina.

The patient should be at once referred for a gynaecological opinion. She should be closely observed pending transfer.

Faintness

The patient should lie down; facilities should be available for her to rest under observation for between one and two hours if necessary. If the faintness is not relieved by recumbency and simple analgesics for pain relief, removal of the IUD should be considered. If the device is removed, return for fitting of a smaller IUD or for advice on other methods of contraception should be suggested.

Bleeding; Uterine Cramps; Pelvic Pain

Bleeding, uterine cramps or pelvic pain experienced immediately following IUD fitting are usually trivial. If significant bleeding or continuous pain unrelieved by simple analgesics continues after an hour or two's rest and observation, prompt transfer to hospital for a gynaecological opinion is indicated.

Immediate Expulsion

The patient should be refitted with another IUD which is less likely to be expelled (e.g. a device known to have a low expulsion rate such as the Antigon). Refitting a larger device may reduce the likelihood of expulsion but complaints concerning an increase in bleeding or pelvic pain are often made.

If a second IUD is immediately expelled serious consideration should be given to using an alternative method of contraception.

Summary of the IUD Fitting Procedure

1. Discuss procedure with patient
2. Place patient in a comfortable position
3. Speculum examination of vagina and cervix
4. Take cervical smear
5. Bimanual examination of uterus
6. Reinsert bivalve vaginal speculum
7. Clean the cervix
8. Attach tenaculum to anterior or lateral vaginal aspect of cervix and bring uterus into line with cervical canal
9. Sound the uterus
10. Place IUD in inserter
11. Fit the IUD
12. Remove the inserter
13. Trim the IUD tail
14. Watch patient for possible immediate post-fitting complications
15. Provide patient with instructions for checking the presence of the IUD; advice regarding possible symptoms; and arrangements for follow-up.

FOLLOW-UP OF IUD PATIENTS

Introduction

The problems associated with IUD use are:

1. Irregular bleeding and pain
2. Expulsion

3. Pregnancy
4. Pelvic inflammatory disease
5. Perforation

Most patient complaints are concerned with some aspect of bleeding irregularity and the experience of uterine cramps or pelvic pain. Pregnancy, pelvic inflammatory disease and perforation are generally considered to be the most serious occurrences when an IUD is being used but they are not the most common.

Function of Follow-Up

The purpose in undertaking a follow-up examination of the IUD patient is to check that the IUD is correctly in place, to assess the patient's health and to deal with any side effects reported or requests for assistance made by the patient. Patients who do not attend for follow-up will be exposing themselves to an additional risk of pregnancy if an unnoticed displacement of the IUD has occurred.

Frequency of Follow-Up

If problems are anticipated with a specific patient, the first follow-up visit should take place within a week of fitting. In cases of an uneventful fitting the first follow-up visit is conveniently undertaken after the patient's next menstrual period — that is, between five and six weeks after fitting.

If bleeding, pain, cramp or complete or partial expulsion occur they are most likely to happen in the first few weeks following the IUD fitting. It is therefore desirable to schedule a follow-up visit about three months after the fitting has taken place. Timing of subsequent follow-up visits will depend upon the circumstances of the individual user and the resources available for the provision of a follow-up service. In addition to the early follow-up visit an annual consultation is desirable.

COMPLAINTS BY PATIENT AT FOLLOW-UP VISIT

Missed Period

This is unusual among IUD users. Check the presence of the IUD tail and consider the possibility that the patient is pregnant.

Sudden Commencement of Intermenstrual Spotting

If this occurs in a previously asymptomatic IUD user, refer to a gynaecologist. The cause needs to be ascertained.

Irregular and Persistent Bleeding

If this problem persists, check for anaemia. If patient is anaemic (i.e. haemoglobin below 11g/100 ml) remove the IUD. If not anaemic but bleeding continues, refer the patient to a gynaecologist. This condition requires diagnosis and treatment.

Irregular Bleeding and Pain

Consider a possible ectopic pregnancy. If the history is strongly suggestive — a missed or abnormally scanty period, brown vaginal discharge, breast tenderness and severe lower abdominal or pelvic pain more on one side — the patient should be referred promptly to hospital *before* a pelvic examination is attempted.

During the first few weeks after fitting some uterine cramps or low backache may be experienced but these side effects normally become less as time goes on. Menstrual periods are nearly always heavier and rather longer following the fitting of an IUD. Mid-cycle spotting or brown discharge is common. Changes in bleeding patterns are difficult to evaluate owing to the problems in estimating the actual amount of blood lost. The majority of investigators report only those cases in which this side effect is troublesome enough to necessitate removal of the device and the severity of bleeding is not the only factor determining whether or not the device is removed. The user's attitude and the approach of the attending doctor play an important part in the rate of IUD removal following a complaint of bleeding or pain. Nevertheless removal following such complaints is the most common reason for IUD discontinuation. Unlike the risk of expulsion, which decrease with duration of use, removal for bleeding or pain remains a relatively constant risk whilst the device is being worn.

A description of the rate of bleeding/pain removal by type of device and age/parity of the IUD acceptor is given in Section II of this manual.

Cause

Apart from the slight trauma at the time of insertion a likely explanation for the occurrence of bleeding and pain is that the size and shape of the device is not compatible with the size and shape of the uterus. The rate of removal for complaints of this nature does increase with the larger sizes of IUD models. It has been demonstrated that multiparous women tend to have fewer bleeding and pain removals than women wearing the same device but who have had no confinements. Obviously an IUD is more easily accommodated in the bulkier uterus of a woman who has had several pregnancies.

It is known that fibrinolysis is enhanced by the presence of an IUD and this and reduced coagulability of the menstrual loss increases the amount of bleeding. It has also been suggested that encrustation with calcium deposits on the surface of the device may contribute to the bleeding problem either because the surface of the device becomes rough and irritates the endometrial lining or because the deposition of calcium interferes in some way with the mechanism of blood clotting.

IUDs containing progesterone are known to be associated with some increase in the frequency of bleeding. The local hormone effect presumably interferes with the normal menstrual sloughing and passage of the endometrium.

Treatment

At the time of IUD fitting, the patient should be warned to expect a certain amount of bleeding immediately following fitting and that subsequent menstrual periods will be heavier than usual. She should be reassured that this is a normal reaction. Care must be taken when reassuring the patient about the appearance of these symptoms that she is not made to feel hesitant about returning for a check visit if the symptoms become unacceptable to her.

Various forms of treatment have been tried for bleeding complaints but none has proved entirely successful. Harmless measures include ascorbic acid, calcium, vitamins (especially vitamins D and K) and ferrous sulphate, as well as a progestogen in the second half of the menstrual cycle. It has been shown that oral administration of the fibrinolysis inhibitor aminocaproic acid will reduce the increased blood loss due to an IUD, but aminocaproic acid is unpleasant to take and the effects of prolonged administration are unknown.

Provided the patient is not becoming anaemic, some reassurance from the doctor may reinforce the patient's motivation to continue wearing the IUD.

An analgesic may be given at the time of fitting to women susceptible to pain — particularly the nulliparous or low-parity patient. Analgesics are also recommended for uterine cramps or low backache which may occur in the first few weeks following IUD fitting.

Heavy Bleeding Accompanied by Clots and Uterine Cramps

This may be an abortion. Examine the patient and refer her to a specialist if necessary.

Painful Periods

If dysmenorrhoea develops soon after IUD fitting, the problem should settle down. If the condition persists of gets worse or if it arises *de novo* in a patient who has had an IUD for some months, consider possible gynaecological causes such as pelvic inflammatory disease or endometriosis. If no other cause than the IUD can be detected, replacement by a smaller device less likely to give pain should be considered.

Lower Abdominal or Pelvic Pain or Cramps

Check for:

1. Pyrexia
2. Uterine tenderness and pain on moving the uterus, adnexal swelling and tenderness or tenderness in the pouch of Douglas.
3. Abdominal signs of peritonitis.

Consider the possibility of:

1. Pelvic inflammatory disease
2. Perforation (and peritonitis)
3. Ectopic pregnancy

If one of these conditions is suspected, do not attempt to remove the IUD but refer at once to a gynaecologist. If there are no abnormal abdominal or pelvic signs it may be reasonable to prescribe a simple analgesic and review the situation the following day. If this is done, the patient must report at once if the pain gets worse or new symptoms such as nausea or vomiting develop.

If the patient has used an IUD for some time without trouble the onset of lower abdominal or pelvic pain should be taken very seriously

Husband Complains that He 'Feels' IUD

1. Check whether the device has become displaced or is partially or completely extruded into the vagina.
2. If the tails are long they may be trimmed.
3. Remember that the husband may have a reason for avoiding intercourse that he has not revealed to his spouse.

ABNORMAL FINDINGS AT THE FOLLOW-UP VISIT

At each follow-up visit all side effects reported as having occurred since the previous visit should be recorded. The cervix should be visualised to confirm the presence of the IUD tail. Signs of pelvic inflammatory disease or a possible pregnancy should be sought by bimanual examination.

Absent Tails

The presence of the IUD tail should be checked by palpation; they are sometimes palpable when they are not easy to see. The IUD may have turned in the uterus and wound up the tail. If the tail is absent, the presence of the device can be ascertained by inserting a sterile sound and gently probing the canal and uterine cavity. This sounding may precipitate bleeding and will often be uncomfortable for the patient. An X-ray examination will indicate the presence of the IUD in the pelvis provided the device contains barium or other metal. In general it will not confirm that the device is wholly within the uterus. Hysterosalpingography may be required to localise the device accurately but is of course contra-indicated if a pregnancy is suspected.

Ultrasound B-scan may be used to localise an IUD accurately whether or not the patient is pregnant but the equipment is usually available only in hospitals.

If the IUD cannot be found, consider:

1.   Expulsion
2.   Pregnancy
3.   Perforation

IUD is Partly Expelled from the Uterus

Check for pregnancy and if not pregnant remove IUD by slow traction on the tail. Consider the refitting of another IUD.

IUD is Not Present in Uterus, Pelvis or Abdomen

Check that the patient is not pregnant. Another IUD can be fitted if a pregnancy is not suspected.

Fragmentation of the Device in situ

This may be diagnosed by an abdominal X-ray, or part of the fragmented device may be passed *per vaginam*. The patient should be referred for a gynaecological opinion.

Cervical Erosion

An asymptomatic erosion does not require treatment if a cervical smear is normal. If the smear shows only cervicitis but the patient complains of a discharge, the erosion can be treated with cautery or the cryoprobe with the device *in situ*. It is unlikely to heal as rapidly or completely as it will if the device is removed for two months.

Adnexal Mass

If an adnexal mass is felt, the patient should be referred for a gynaecological opinion. If the mass is tender it could be an ectopic gestation or pelvic inflammatory disease. Excessive palpation should be avoided and a gynaecological opinion obtained at once.

IUD REMOVAL

Removal of the device is usually accomplished by gentle traction on the tail attached to the device. If there is any resistance the cervix should be dilated to Hegar 4 or 5 before further traction is applied.

An IUD removal can nearly always be conducted as an out-patient procedure but sometimes admission to hospital and a general anaestheti may be necessary. A feeling of faintness is not uncommon at the time of removal. If this occurs the patient should rest under observation for a short time.

If any part of the tail can be located, use small sponge-holding forceps, polyp forceps or Spencer-Wells forceps to grasp it and then remove the IUD by gentle slow traction. Devices without tail threads (e.g. some Antigons) and devices from which the tail has become detached or drawn up into the uterus may be removed using a Gräfenberg hook, designed for the purpose.

If difficulty is encountered, specialist advice should be sought.

EXPULSION

The rate of expulsion has been reported as ranging between 2 per cent and 20 per cent during the first year of use depending upon the device concerned, the characteristics of the IUD acceptor and the clinic attended. When the bio-engineers became interested in the developmen of a 'non-expellable' device, it was not surprising that a marked drop in the incidence of expulsion was obtained. Nor was it surprising that there were reports of increased perforation rates with the new 'fundal-seeking' devices they designed. The risk of expulsion has not ye been eliminated.

Nulliparous acceptors and women below the age of thirty are at greater risk of expulsion than older, parous women. The overall risk of expulsion is highest in the first three months after fitting of the device, when about 50 per cent of all expulsions occur. Very few expulsions occur after the first year of use and for this reason it is particularly important that a follow-up check visit is undertaken shortly after fitting and again at the end of the first year of use. The incidence of partial expulsion (i.e. the displacement of part of the device into the cervix or vagina) is probably higher than the incidence of complete expulsion. This is a particular problem because the partial expulsion is more likely to go unnoticed by the woman, though the consort may detect an unusual sensation.

A detailed description of the rate of expulsion by type of device an age and parity of the IUD acceptor is given in Section II of this manua

Cause

The anatomical features of the uterus, the fitting technique and the timing of insertion all affect the incidence of expulsion. The likelihood of a device being expelled from the uterus depends on how closely the device configuration fits the size and shape of the uterine cavity and on the extent to which the device is able to absorb uterine contractions. Linear devices should be loaded into the introducer immediately before use to prevent loss of IUD 'memory' or there is an increased risk of expulsion. At the time of fitting it is important to ensure that the device is placed entirely within the uterine cavity so that no part of the IUD (except the threads) is left in the cervical canal.

Devices fitted in the early post-abortum and post-partum period and during menses are more prone to immediate expulsion because the cervix at such times is more relaxed. A follow-up visit, preferably within one month but no later than three months, should be strictly observed if fittings are undertaken during menses or after delivery:

Expulsion Reported by the Patient

If pregnancy can be excluded, another IUD may be fitted using a device which is known to have a low rate of expulsion (see Section II).

ACCIDENTAL PREGNANCY

The presence of a device correctly placed within the uterine cavity does not entirely preclude the occurrence of an unintended pregnancy. To determine the reasons why an IUD can fail to prevent a pregnancy, it would be necessary to have a clearer understanding of how the IUD exerts its contraceptive effect than is at present available. Experience and skill in fitting the IUD will also affect the risk of pregnancy. An unnoticed expulsion, perforation of the device through the uterine wall or displacement of the device into the cervix will increase exposure to the risk of accidental pregnancy.

A description of the pregnancy rates by type of device and age and parity of the IUD acceptor is given in Section II of this manual.

Patient Presents with a Missed Period

The following steps should be taken:

1. Insert a speculum.
2. Check for IUD tail.
3. Examine the pelvis bimanually.
4. Verify pregnancy by a urine pregnancy diagnosis test.
5. It is reasonable to remove the device if the maturity of the pregnancy is less than three months, the strings are visible, and there is no undue resistance to traction on them. Some feel that

this is an unwise manoeuvre to perform in a family planning clinic or a doctor's surgery, as it can be followed by heavy bleeding.

6. If the IUD cannot be detected, do *not* probe the uterus.
7. Accept that the IUD may or may not be present in the uterus.
8. If the patient is pregnant, notify the family doctor informing him that location of the IUD is not known and giving details of the IUD concerned.
9. A careful search should be made at the time of delivery and if the IUD is not found, the patient should be X-rayed after the confinement.

Outcome of Pregnancy

Two out of every three pregnancies associated with IUD use are reported as occurring with the device *in situ*. If the IUD is placed where it interferes with the growing foetus a spontaneous abortion will result but many pregnancies continue normally, ending with a normal full-term live birth.

Between 1972 and 1976 the United Kingdom IUD network received reports of 574 pregnancies associated with the use of a wide variety of IUDs. Table I provides details of the 466 pregnancies where the outcome

TABLE I: Known Outcome of Pregnancies Reported between 1972 and 1976. University of Exeter, Family Planning Research Unit

	TOTAL		Lippes Loop A	Lippes Loop B	Lippes Loop C	Lippes Loop D	Saf-T-Coil Standard	Gravigard	Gyne T	Wing Antigon	Other
Total* pregnancies where outcome is known	466		15	9	48	29	35	130	5	20	175**
Live birth	126	(27%)	6 (40%)	3 (33%)	14 (29%)	11 (38%)	11 (31%)	37 (28%)	2 (40%)	5 (25%)	37 (21%)
Still birth	5	(1%)	–	–	1 (2%)	–	–	1 (1%)	1 (20%)	–	2 (1%)
Therapeutic abortion	191	(41%)	5 (33%)	1 (11%)	17 (35%)	11 (38%)	18 (51%)	61 (47%)	1 (20%)	6 (30%)	71 (41%)
Spontaneous abortion	119	(26%)	3 (20%)	3 (33%)	12 (25%)	5 (17%)	5 (14%)	27 (21%)	1 (20%)	6 (30%)	57 (33%)
Ectopic	25	(5%)	1 (7%)	2 (22%)	4 (8%)	2 (7%)	1 (3%)	4 (3%)	–	3 (15%)	8 (4%)

* A total 574 pregnancies have been reported but some of these are continuing at the time of writing and the outcome of others is not known. This table is confined to *known* pregnancy outcome.

** The Dalkon Shield provided 157 of these pregnancies but this device has not been treated separately as it is no longer generally available. (See 'IUD and Mortality Risk'.)

of pregnancy was ascertained. All these pregnancies are the result of conceptions which occurred at a time when the IUD was believed to be *in situ* by the patient concerned.

It is not surprising that most of these pregnancies end in a therapeutic abortion as these patients have already indicated that a pregnancy would cause difficulties by accepting an IUD. Care should be taken in generalising from the figures for those devices which provide data on only a few pregnancies. It should also be noted that Table I does not provide evidence of a pregnancy (failure) rate as some devices have been fitted in much larger numbers than others.

Prognosis

The patient who learns that she has become pregnant when wearing an IUD is likely to react in one of three ways:

1. The patient does not want this pregnancy and asks for advice about therapeutic abortion.
2. The patient is unsure and wants further counselling concerning the pregnancy and its possible outcome.
3. The patient wishes to continue with the pregnancy.

If the patient asks for a therapeutic abortion she should be referred appropriately. If a vaginal examination is performed or an attempt made to remove the IUD in these circumstances it could possibly be construed as an attempt to procure an illegal abortion.

If the patient wishes to continue with the pregnancy she should be warned of the possibility of spontaneous abortion and should receive specialist antenatal care and have a hospital confinement. At the time of delivery (or miscarriage) the whereabouts of the IUD should be ascertained — some cases of IUD retention *in utero* after delivery have been reported.

Suspected Pregnancy

If the IUD tail is not visible and there is doubt about the pregnancy, the patient should be referred to a hospital for examination. An X-ray should not be taken but ultrasound techniques can be used to locate the IUD.

Spontaneous Abortion and Full-term births

The majority of spontaneous abortions occur in the first trimester of pregnancy irrespective of the IUD model being worn. A comparison of the incidence of spontaneous abortion and full term births is interesting as it demonstrates the outcome of pregnancy among those *not* seeking therapeutic abortion. The incidence of 'spontaneous' abortion may well include a number of induced abortion cases and for this reason the figures given for spontaneous abortion may be inflated. This factor may be partly responsible for the slight variation between different devices. A number of the recorded spontaneous abortions are believed to have been 'helped' by the IUD user and occasionally by the doctor examining the patient at follow-up visits. Nevertheless, it would appear that a patient wishing to continue with a pregnancy has about an even chance of going to full term. (See Table I.)

Two septic mid-trimester abortions have been reported in the United Kingdom study. Both patients were wearing a Dalkon Shield (a device which is no longer generally available) but both were atypical cases. In one, gonorrhoea was also present and in the other there was a suspicion that the patient had herself attempted to induce an abortion. The risk of a septic abortion among United Kingdom IUD users is very low but this condition should never be entirely ruled out when caring for the pregnant IUD patient.

Removal or Expulsion of IUD During Pregnancy

Where the removal of the device without difficulty is possible early in pregnancy there is an increased probability that the pregnancy will go to term (see Table II). Removal of the IUD as a routine measure among pregnant IUD patients should depend on three basic criteria:

1. The pregnancy is in the first trimester.
2. The tail of the device is visible at the external os.
3. The device is easy to remove *at the first attempt.*

Some doctors believe that even if all these conditions are met it is unwise to remove an IUD outside hospital premises. If heavy bleeding occurs at the time of removal, this can be coped with more easily in the hospital environment. Removal of an IUD later than the first trimester should not be attempted. The advice of a gynaecologist should be sought in such cases.

The advisability of removing the device after a pregnancy has been diagnosed will depend on the IUD model being worn, the stage of pregnancy and the woman's feelings toward continuing with the pregnancy. It is recommended that a woman who is believed to be pregnant with an IUD *in situ* should be informed of the consequences of removing the device or of leaving it alone. In either event the progress of the pregnancy should be very carefully followed.

Ectopic Pregnancy

Also recorded among the 466 pregnancies in the United Kingdom IUD study are 25 ectopic pregnancies. The 1:19 ratio of ectopic pregnancies to the total number of pregnancies among IUD users is

TABLE II: Comparison of Spontaneous Abortions and Live Births among IUD Patients where the IUD was known to be Present at the Delivery or known to have been Expelled or Removed in Early Pregnancy 1972–6

	Total	Lippes Loop A	Lippes Loop B	Lippes Loop C	Lippes Loop D	Saf-T-Coil Standard	Gravigard	Gyne T	Wing Antigon	Other
Total relevant pregnancies with IUD in situ	132	4	4	13	10	9	38	2	4	48
Live birth	56 (42%)	3 (75%)	1 (25%)	4 (31%)	6 (60%)	5 (56%)	18 (47%)	1 (50%)	2 (50%)	16 (33%)
Spontaneous abortion	76 (58%)	1 (25%)	3 (75%)	9 (69%)	4 (40%)	4 (44%)	20 (53%)	1 (50%)	2 (50%)	32 (67%)
Total relevant pregnancies with IUD removed or expelled early in pregnancy	35	4	–	4	2	4	13	–	2	6
Live birth	25 (71%)	3 (75%)	–	4 (100%)	1 (50%)	4 (100%)	9 (69%)	–	–	4 (67%)
Spontaneous abortion	10 (29%)	1 (25%)	–	–	1 (50%)	–	4 (31%)	–	2 (100%)	2 (33%)

slightly higher than that reported in the largest American study. Discussions continue concerning the part an IUD may be playing in relation to ectopic pregnancy. Some claim that the IUD is associated with a reduction in the incidence of ectopic pregnancy but others claim the reverse. One point is clear and not disputed — the IUD user who is pregnant with the IUD *in situ* is much more likely to have an ectopic pregnancy than the pregnant patient who is not wearing an IUD. For this reason, it is essential that the possibility of an ectopic pregnancy is carefully checked whenever a patient wearing an IUD becomes pregnant. Additional care should also be taken whenever the IUD patient complains of sudden abdominal pain or reports a late or missed period.

Pregnancy and Perforation

A pregnancy may occur when an undiagnosed perforation of the device has occurred. Two cases of perforation associated with pregnancy were reported in the United Kingdom study. A live birth was the outcome in one case and in the other case a premature birth occurred at 28 weeks and the baby died after 12 hours. In both cases the device was located in the peritoneal cavity following delivery.

If the device is not found at the time of delivery and there is no knowledge of an expulsion having taken place during pregnancy, a careful examination should be undertaken to ascertain that a perforation has not occurred or that the device is still in the uterus.

Foetal Abnormality

No evidence has been obtained in the United Kingdom study which suggests that the IUD has a teratogenic effect on the foetus. Full-term babies born to mothers wearing an IUD during pregnancy are no more likely to have foetal abnormalities than babies born to mothers not wearing an IUD.

Mortality

No cases of death following a complication of pregnancy associated with any IUD model have been reported in the Exeter IUD network. Two deaths among IUD wearers have been recorded in recent years but neither of these were associated with pregnancy. In both cases death was related to chronic infection; in one case this was introduced either *via* a track in the cervix caused by forceps or *via* the lining of the uterus in the other, the patient was undergoing steroid therapy and PID was being masked.

Information from studies outside the United Kingdom indicate that most deaths linked with IUD use are associated with pregnancy. Since intrauterine devices were first introduced for general use in the United States (1965) there have been thirty-nine reported deaths which are believed to have occurred as a result of IUD use. Pregnancy complications accounted for twenty-one of these deaths, with thirteen associated with one IUD model — the Dalkon Shield. Between 1965 and 1974 approximately 8,795,000 intrauterine devices were distributed. It is estimated that on the basis of these figures the mortality risk among IUD users is in the region of 1 to 10 per million woman years of use. This risk is of the same order as the risk among women taking oral contraceptives.

The IUD is not without its imperfections but present evidence suggests it provides a relatively safe form of contraception when compared to other methods currently available.

PELVIC INFLAMMATORY DISEASE (PID)

Estimating the incidence of pelvic inflammatory disease is difficult because of uncertainty surrounding the diagnosis and reporting of this complaint. It is known that the incidence of PID among IUD users is higher than that among non-IUD users. The diagnosis of PID is almost entirely dependent upon clinical judgement and this makes assessments of incidence unreliable for comparative purposes. Most reports concerning PID among IUD users indicate numbers of cases which require removal of the device although these may account for only a proportion of the total number of IUD patients experiencing this condition. In the United Kingdom study about one case of PID is reported for every 250 IUD fittings each year although this rate does vary according to the device model concerned — from 1:104 with the Gravigard (Copper 7), to 1:385 with the Lippes Loop B. In about half of the cases of pelvic inflammatory disease with a device *in situ* reported in the United Kingdom, removal of the device is undertaken, either at once or after initiation of antibiotic treatment.

TABLE III: Reported Cases of Pelvic Inflammatory Disease. University of Exeter, Family Planning Research Unit. 1972—6

	Lippes Loop B	Lippes Loop C	Lippes Loop D	Saf-T-Coil	Gravigard	Gyne T	Wing Antigon
Treatment only (no removal)	—	7 (33%)	2 (29%)	4 (33%)	21 (30%)	3 (75%)	3 (60%)
Treatment accompanied by IUD removal	—	11 (52%)	5 (71%)	7 (58%)	41 (59%)	1 (25%)	2 (40%)
Treatment not known	1 (100%)	3 (15%)	—	1 (9%)	8 (11%)	—	—
TOTAL CASES	1	21	7	12	70	4	5
Rate per 1,000 fittings per year	2.6	5.1	2.9	3.6	9.6	3.9	8.0

Some doctors treat mild inflammatory reactions with antibiotics while the device remains in the uterus. Most doctors will remove an IUD in the presence of a gonococcal infection. This is based on the belief that the presence of an IUD may encourage the infection to ascend into the uterus and tubes. It has been suggested that copper carrying devices have a bactericidal effect which provides some protection against ascending gonococcal infection but it is unlikely that concentrations of copper sufficient to have any therapeutic value are achieved.

Table III gives information concerning reports of PID among users of IUDs fitted in clinics cooperating in the United Kingdom IUD network.

PERFORATION

The incidence of perforation appears to be related to the type of IUD model being fitted, the condition of the uterus and cervix and the skill of the person responsible for fitting the IUD. Table IV provides crude rates of perforation for some of the IUDs discussed in this manual. Approximately one perforation in every 500 fittings is reported among Lippes Loop users. The ratio of perforations to fittings with the newer devices such as the Gyne T (Copper T) and the Gravigard (Copper 7) is said to be approximately 1:1,500. Certain devices have been associated with unusually high rates of perforation — the M device and the older model of the Birnberg Bow — and are for this reason no longer generally available.

TABLE IV: Crude Perforation Rates per 1,000 IUD First Fittings 1972—6

All devices:	0.90*
Gravigard	0.62**
Gyne T	0.67
Lippes Loop C	1.23
Lippes Loop D	3.37
All Lippes Loop Models	2.0

*   This ratio represents the crude perforation rate per 1,000 first fittings.
**   Includes cervical perforations.

Between 1972 and 1976, no perforations were recorded with the following devices: Lippes Loop A (243 fittings); Lippes Loop B (422 fittings); Saf-T-Coil (2,737 fittings); Antigon (827 fittings).

Cause

Nearly all perforations start at the time of IUD fitting. Perforations most commonly occur when fitting an IUD into an acutely anteflexed or retroverted uterus or where fitting has been attempted soon after delivery. Many doctors consider that careful sounding to confirm the position and depth of the uterus should always be undertaken before IUD fitting and undue force should never be used to negotiate the cervical canal. Where resistance is felt the sound or IUD inserter should be removed and either another attempt made after a review of the position of the uterus or the IUD fitting abandoned altogether. Most doctors use a tenaculum to draw the uterus into the axis of the cervical canal to permit easier IUD fitting and to reduce the possibility of uterine or cervical perforation.

The most usual form of perforation is through the wall of the body of the uterus but cervical perforations have also been reported. These cervical perforations are confined to the newer IUDs such as the Gravigard, in the United Kingdom series. This may be due to the design of the IUD which results in the vertical stem of the '7' being driven into the 'wall' of the cervical canal if the device is expelled by the uterus. Studies have reported cervical perforations with other devices and a note should be made that such perforations are possible even though the incidence of the complication is very low.

Perforation and Pregnancy

If perforation has occurred the patient is no longer protected against pregnancy and conception may occur. As a result many perforations are found to be associated with an unwanted pregnancy.

Treatment

In cases of suspected or known perforation, the patient should be referred to a gynaecologist. In most cases of perforation, the device tail is no longer visible at the external os but even if the tail is visible and perforation is suspected the IUD should not be removed without previous consultation with a specialist.

SECTION II

Part 1: THE IUD USER
Part 2: THE IUD MODEL

PART 1: THE IUD USER

This part of Section II contains data relating to patients with the following characteristics.

1.	Nulliparous	6.	High age
2.	Parous	7.	Low age and low parity
3.	Low parity	8.	Low age and high parity
4.	High parity	9.	High age and low parity
5.	Low age	10.	High age and high parity

USE-EFFECTIVENESS RATES

In interpreting the rates described, the following points should be borne in mind:

1. The rates are based on general experience during the period 1972—6 in the United Kingdom. They do not represent strictly comparable findings from randomly distributed IUD fittings in a carefully controlled clinical trial. They provide general information concerning IUD experience in the United Kingdom.
2. The rates represent the average findings from twenty centres in the United Kingdom.
3. Unless otherwise stated, the rates are calculated by the Tietze/Potter life-table approach at one year of use.

Definitions

The life-table approach used in the calculation of net event and closure rates for the devices described in this Section gives the probability of a defined risk occurring in or before the nth month following fitting of the device. It also takes into consideration the possibility of other, alternative risks within the same period.

After the fitting of an IUD, the follow-up of that fitting must end in one of five outcomes:

1. The wearer is continuing to wear the IUD successfully.
2. A pregnancy occurs whilst the wearer believes the IUD to be in place.
3. Expulsion of the device occurs.
4. The device is removed.
5. The wearer's progress is no longer followed.

The following definitions relate to these five possible outcomes:

Events	Pregnancy, removal, expulsion, release from follow-up, loss to follow-up.
Closures	Events not followed by refitting of an IUD. Release from follow-up and loss to follow-up are included in the definition of closures.
Pregnancies	Pregnancies are categorised as the outcome when the IUD is known or believed to be *in situ* at the time of conception. If the patient has noticed an expulsion of the IUD or the IUD has been removed before the conception date, then subsequent pregnancy is not strictly an IUD failure. For statistical purposes, conception is taken as having occurred fourteen days after the last menstrual period. The 'event' of pregnancy is assessed as having occurred on that date.
Low Pregnancy Rate	Less than 2 per 100 women per year.
Moderate Pregnancy Rate	Between 2.0 and 4.9 per 100 women per year.
High Pregnancy Rate	5.0 and over per 100 women per year.
Expulsion	An expulsion occurs when the IUD is wholly or partly expelled from the uterus even if subsequent removal is necessary. The expulsion may or may not be noticed by the patient. For statistical purposes the mid-date between the discovery of the IUD absence and the date of the last occasion when the IUD was known to be *in situ* is taken as the date of the 'event'.
	Un-noticed expulsions should not be confused with pregnancies where the site of the IUD is not determined (i.e. when the whereabouts of the IUD are not known at the time of conception). Should a pregnancy occur, even if the investigator later discovers that an expulsion has taken place, the event is still classified as a pregnancy with the presence of the IUD not determined.
Low Expulsion Rate	Up to 5.0 per 100 women per year.
Moderate Expulsion Rate	Between 5.1 and 9.9 per 100 women per year.
High Expulsion Rate	10.0 and over per 100 women per year.
Removal	There is a specific statistical category for removal of the IUD following complaint of bleeding and/or pain attributed to the IUD. Removals for other medical reasons include all those following complaint of physical

discomfort by wife or husband attributed to the IUD even if the examining doctor considers there are no medical grounds for such a complaint.

Removal at the doctor's choice occurs when the examining doctor removes the device because of IUD distortion as seen by X-ray, or when a routine change is thought necessary. Removal of the IUD in order to conceive is a final category.

Low Bleeding/Pain Removal Rate	Up to 5.0 per 100 women per year.
Moderate Bleeding/Pain Removal Rate	Between 5.1 and 9.9 per 100 women per year.
High Bleeding/Pain Removal Rate	10.0 and over per 100 women per year.

Release From Follow-Up

A woman is 'released' when she is transferred to the care of another clinic or doctor outside the areas covered by this study.

Loss to Follow-Up

A woman is considered 'lost' if she is six or more months overdue for a clinic visit and no subsequent information has been received from the patient.

DEVICE	PREGNANCY	EXPULSION	REMOVAL FOR BLEEDING/PAIN
Lippes Loop A	HIGH At least 5.4 (6 month rate)	HIGH At least 13.2 (6 month rate)	MODERATE At least 9.8 (6 month rate)
Saf-T-Coil (25SX)	MODERATE At least 3.2 (4 month rate)	HIGH At least 10.3 (4 month rate)	MODERATE At least 8.3 (4 month rate)
Gravigard (Copper 7)	MODERATE 2.0 ± 0.3	HIGH 15.3 ± 0.8	MODERATE 8.5 ± 0.6
Gyne T (Copper T)	LOW At least 0.7 (6 month rate)	MODERATE At least 7.3 (6 month rate)	MODERATE At least 6.0 (6 month rate)

Based on one year of use unless otherwise stated. Figures represent net event rates (with S.E.) per 100 users, with at least 100 women remaining in the study.

DEVICE INFORMATION	GENERAL CONSIDERATIONS
1. Above average pregnancy, expulsion and removal rates. 2. Over 75 per cent of patients refuse another IUD after experiencing a pregnancy, expulsion or removal.	The data for the Lippes Loop A, Saf-T-Coil and Gyne T (Copper T) are minimal estimates being based on only four or six months of use. The rates for a full year of use are likely to be proportionately higher. *Pregnancy:* From this data, the copper carrying devices yield the lowest pregnancy rates for this category of IUD acceptor. The rate given for the Lippes Loop A is very high and it appears likely that the annual rate for the Saf-T-Coil 25SX will also be high. The Gravigard (Copper 7) is the most popular IUD for this category of patient and represents 85 per cent of fittings. This device has a pregnancy rate in nulliparae similar to that found among parous women. Though the Gyne T has a comparatively low pregnancy rate in nulliparous women the rate at six months is higher than that among other groups of women wearing this device.
1. Above average pregnancy, expulsion and removal rates. 2. Most accept another IUD after an expulsion but not after a pregnancy or removal.	
1. Average pregnancy rate; above average expulsion rate; below average removal rate. 2. Small increase in pregnancy rate, sharp decrease in expulsion rate and gradual decrease in removal rate during the second year of use. 3. Most accept another IUD after expulsion but not after a pregnancy or removal.	*Expulsion:* There is a consistently high expulsion rate in nulliparae with all devices, compared to the experience of parous women. Most of these expulsions occur in the early months of use. *Removal:* With the exception of the Gravigard device (Copper 7), the removal rates for bleeding and/or pain tend to be higher among nulliparous patients than among parous patients.
1. Below average pregnancy rate; average expulsion rate; above average removal rate. 2. Most accept another IUD after expulsion but not after a pregnancy or removal.	*Conclusion:* About 20 per cent of all IUD fittings in the clinic network are in nulliparous patients. The data collected suggest that this category of patient is not the best IUD candidate, but if an IUD is fitted the most appropriate devices are the Gravigard and the Gyne T.

DEVICE	PREGNANCY	EXPULSION	REMOVAL FOR BLEEDING/PAIN
Lippes Loop B	LOW 1.3 ± 0.7	MODERATE 8.5 ± 1.7	MODERATE 9.7 ± 1.8
Lippes Loop C	LOW 1.2 ± 0.2	MODERATE 7.3 ± 0.5	HIGH 12.2 ± 0.6
Lippes Loop D	LOW 1.5 ± 0.3	MODERATE 5.1 ± 0.6	HIGH 10.0 ± 0.8
Saf-T-Coil (Standard)	LOW 1.2 ± 0.2	MODERATE 9.2 ± 0.6	HIGH 13.9 ± 0.8

Based on one year of use. Figures represent net event rates (with S.E.) per 100 users, with at least 100 women remaining in the study during the twelfth month.

DEVICE INFORMATION	GENERAL CONSIDERATIONS
1. Average pregnancy, expulsion and removal rates. 2. Most accept another IUD after expulsion but not after a pregnancy or removal.	The parous woman is considered to be the ideal IUD candidate especially when the IUD is being used for the purpose of spacing pregnancies. *Pregnancy:* Some risk of pregnancy still remains but this is generally very low for this category of patient. There is little to choose between the devices listed with the exception of the Gyne T which has a particularly low pregnancy rate. The Gyne T has the disadvantage of requiring removal at the end of two years of use but many feel that this period of use could safely be extended.
1. Average pregnancy rate; below average expulsion rate; above average removal rate. 2. Constant pregnancy rate, sharp decrease in expulsion rate and gradual decrease in removal rate in second year of use. 3. Most accept another IUD after expulsion but not after a pregnancy or removal.	*Expulsion:* The devices with the lowest expulsion rates are the Lippes Loop D and the Gyne T. There is not much to choose between the other devices which demonstrate an expulsion rate between 7.3 and 9.2 per 100 women during the first year of use. Rates calculated beyond the first year of use indicate that a decrease in the rate of expulsion occurs (with most devices demonstrating a sharp decrease in the incidence of this event) thereafter.
1. Average pregnancy and removal rates; lower than average expulsion rate. 2. Gradual decrease in pregnancy rate, sharp decrease in expulsion rate and constant rate of removal in second year of use. 3. Most accept another IUD after expulsion but not after a pregnancy or removal.	*Removal:* The Gyne T (Copper T) has the lowest rate of removal following a complaint of bleeding and/or pain among the devices fitted between 1972 and 1976 in the United Kingdom. The Lippes Loop B, Lippes Loop D and the Gravigard also demonstrate removal rates of 10 per cent or less in the first year of use. The rate of removal in the second year of use either gradually decreases or remains constant depending on the IUD model.
1. Average pregnancy and expulsion rates; above average removal rate. 2. Gradual decrease in pregnancy and removal rates and sharp decrease in expulsion rate in second year of use. 3. Most accept another IUD after expulsion but not after a pregnancy or removal.	*continued overleaf*

DEVICE	PREGNANCY	EXPULSION	REMOVAL FOR BLEEDING/PAIN
Gravigard (Copper 7)	MODERATE 2.2 ± 0.2	MODERATE 9.1 ± 0.5	HIGH 10.0 ± 0.5
Gyne T (Copper T)	LOW 0.3 ± 0.2	MODERATE 5.2 ± 0.9	MODERATE 7.4 ± 1.0
Antigon (Wing)	LOW 1.1 ± 0.5	MODERATE 9.1 ± 1.5	HIGH 11.9 ± 1.8
Antigon (Film)	LOW 1.2 ± 0.6	MODERATE 8.9 ± 1.6	HIGH 18.4 ± 2.2

Based on one year of use. Figures represent net event rates (with S.E.) per 100 users, with at least 100 women remaining in the study during the twelfth month.

DEVICE INFORMATION	GENERAL CONSIDERATIONS
1. Above average pregnancy rate; average expulsion and removal rates. 2. Gradual decrease in pregnancy and removal rates and sharp decrease in expulsion rate in second year of use. 3. Most accept another IUD after expulsion but not after pregnancy or removal.	*Conclusion:* The data obtained in the IUD clinic network indicates that of the devices considered for this category of patient the Gyne T appears to be the most successful during the first year of use. The disadvantages of this device at the present time are that there is only limited experience in the United Kingdom of its use, it is said to require replacement at the end of two years and that it is not available on NHS prescription. It is best to use a Lippes Loop D or Gyne T with this category of patient.
1. Below average pregnancy, expulsion and removal rates. 2. Increase in pregnancy rate and gradual decrease in expulsion and removal rates in second year of use. 3. Most accept another device after expulsion but not after a pregnancy or removal.	
1. Average pregnancy and expulsion rates; above average removal rate. 2. Decrease in pregnancy rate, sharp decrease in expulsion rate and constant removal rate in second year of use. 3. Over 75 per cent of patients accept another device after expulsion but most refuse after a pregnancy or removal.	
1. Average pregnancy and expulsion rates; above average removal rate. 2. Decrease in pregnancy and expulsion rates and constant removal rate in second year of use. 3. Most accept another IUD after expulsion but not after a pregnancy or removal.	

DEVICE	PREGNANCY	EXPULSION	REMOVAL FOR BLEEDING/PAIN
Lippes Loop B	LOW 1.7 ± 0.8	HIGH 10.6 ± 2.1	HIGH 10.2 ± 2.1
Lippes Loop C	LOW 1.2 ± 0.2	MODERATE 8.5 ± 0.6	HIGH 12.9 ± 0.8
Lippes Loop D	LOW 1.6 ± 0.4	MODERATE 5.5 ± 0.7	HIGH 10.4 ± 1.0
Saf-T-Coil (Standard)	LOW 1.3 ± 0.3	HIGH 10.5 ± 0.8	HIGH 14.2 ± 0.9

Based on one year of use. Figures represent net event rates (with S.E.) per 100 users, with at least 100 women remaining in the study during the twelfth month.

DEVICE INFORMATION	GENERAL CONSIDERATIONS
1. Average pregnancy, expulsion and removal rates. 2. Most accept another IUD after expulsion but not after a pregnancy or removal.	Taking parity as the distinguishing characteristic and combining the risks of pregnancy, expulsion and removal, the high parity patients (those with parity of 3 or more) are the most successful IUD users and nulliparae the least successful IUD users. Patients of low parity (1 or 2) take up a position midway between these two extreme positions.
1. Average pregnancy, expulsion and removal rates. 2. Constant pregnancy rate, sharp decrease in expulsion rate and gradual decrease in removal rate in second year of use. 3. Most accept another IUD after expulsion but not after a pregnancy or removal.	*Pregnancy:* This category of patient demonstrates low pregnancy rates with all devices with the exception of the Gravigard device which shows a rate slightly above average. The Antigon devices and the Gyne T pregnancy rates are particularly low.
1. Average pregnancy and removal rates; below average expulsion rate. 2. Gradual decrease in pregnancy rate, sharp decrease in expulsion rate and constant rate of removal in second year of use. 3. Most accept another IUD after expulsion but not after a pregnancy or removal.	*Expulsion:* There is little to choose between most of the devices for which rates have been calculated. With the exception of two devices the expulsion rate range is between 8.5 and 10.6 for every 100 women in the first year of use. This is in contrast to the higher parity women (3 and over) who yield rates ranging between 4.0 and 6.6 in the first year of use. The exceptions are the Gyne T with an expulsion rate of 5.3 and the Lippes Loop D with a rate of 5.5.
1. Average pregnancy and expulsion rates; above average removal rate. 2. Gradual decrease in pregnancy, expulsion and removal rates in second year of use. 3. Most accept another IUD after expulsion but not after a pregnancy or removal.	*Removal:* The removal rate ranges between 8.1 and 18.0 for every 100 women at the end of the first year depending on the IUD being used. Most devices are in the narrower range of 10.2 to 12.9 (Lippes Loop B, C, D; Gravigard; and Wing Antigon). The exceptions are the Gyne T with a removal rate of 8.1; the Saf-T-Coil at 14.2; and the Film Antigon at 18.0.

continued overleaf

DEVICE	PREGNANCY	EXPULSION	REMOVAL FOR BLEEDING/PAIN
Gravigard (Copper 7)	MODERATE 2.3 ± 0.3	MODERATE 9.9 ± 0.6	HIGH 10.3 ± 0.6
Gyne T (Copper T)	LOW 0.5 ± 0.3	MODERATE 5.3 ± 1.0	MODERATE 8.1 ± 1.3
Antigon (Wing)	LOW 0.4 ± 0.4	HIGH 10.2 ± 2.0	HIGH 12.6 ± 2.2
Antigon (Film)	LOW 0.8 ± 0.5	MODERATE 9.7 ± 1.9	HIGH 18.0 ± 2.6

Based on one year of use. Figures represent net event rates (with S.E.) per 100 users, with at least 100 women remaining in the study during the twelfth month.

DEVICE INFORMATION

1. Above average pregnancy rate; average expulsion and removal rates.
2. Gradual decrease in pregnancy and removal rates and sharp decrease in expulsion rate in second year of use.
3. Most accept another IUD after expulsion but not after a pregnancy or removal.

---

1. Below average pregnancy, expulsion and removal rates.
2. Increase in pregnancy rate and decrease in expulsion and removal rates in second year of use.
3. Over 75 per cent accept another IUD after expulsion but most refuse after a pregnancy or removal.

---

1. Below average pregnancy rate; average expulsion and removal rates.
2. Increase in pregnancy rate, sharp decrease in expulsion rate and constant removal rate in second year of use.
3. Over 75 per cent accept another IUD after expulsion but most refuse after a pregnancy or removal.

---

1. Below average pregnancy rate; average expulsion rate; very high removal rate.
2. Over 75 per cent accept another IUD after expulsion but most refuse after a pregnancy or removal.

GENERAL CONSIDERATIONS

Conclusion: The pregnancy rates for IUD acceptors with a parity 1 or 2 are similar to those for women with a high parity. The one exception is the rate with the Wing Antigon which has a lower pregnancy rate for those with lower parity.

The expulsion rates are consistently higher for the low parity IUD user than for the high parity acceptor.

Removal rates for the low parity acceptor are also consistently higher than those for the high parity acceptor. The best devices for this group of patients are Lippes Loop C, D, or the Gyne T.

DEVICE	PREGNANCY	EXPULSION	REMOVAL FOR BLEEDING/PAIN
Lippes Loop C	LOW 1.2 ± 0.4	LOW 4.0 ± 0.7	HIGH 10.4 ± 1.2
Lippes Loop D	LOW 1.2 ± 0.5	LOW 4.4 ± 0.9	MODERATE 9.0 ± 1.3
Saf-T-Coil (Standard)	LOW 1.2 ± 0.4	MODERATE 6.0 ± 1.0	HIGH 13.3 ± 1.4

Based on one year of use. Figures represent net event rates (with S.E.) per 100 users, with at least 100 women remaining in the study during the twelfth month.

DEVICE INFORMATION	GENERAL CONSIDERATIONS

DEVICE INFORMATION

1. Average pregnancy, expulsion and removal rates.
2. Constant pregnancy and removal rates and decrease in expulsion rate in second year of use.
3. Over 75 per cent accept another IUD after expulsion but most refuse after a pregnancy or removal.

1. Average pregnancy, expulsion and removal rates.
2. Constant pregnancy and removal rates and sharp decrease in expulsion rate in second year of use.
3. Over 75 per cent accept another IUD after expulsion but most refuse after a pregnancy or removal.

1. Average pregnancy and expulsion rates; above average removal rate.
2. Gradual decrease in pregnancy, expulsion and removal rates in second year of use.
3. Most accept another IUD after expulsion but not after a pregnancy or removal.

GENERAL CONSIDERATIONS

Pregnancy: This category of IUD patient is exposed to a consistently low risk of pregnancy. All devices except one provide a rate at one year of use of 1.6 or less. The exception is the Wing Antigon which demonstrates a higher pregnancy rate.

Expulsion: There is very little to choose between the devices in relation to expulsion. The range is 4.0 to 6.6 per 100 users at the end of the first year of IUD use.

Removal: There is a wider range (6.0 to 13.3) in the removal rate following complaints of bleeding or pain but with most devices the rates are between 8.9 and 10.4 per 100 users at twelve months of use. The exceptions are the Gyne T with a rate of 6.0 and the Saf-T-Coil with a rate of 13.3.

Conclusion: The pregnancy rates for the high parity IUD acceptor are generally similar to those obtained among low parity (1 or 2) IUD acceptors. The one exception is the Wing Antigon which has a higher pregnancy rate among high parity acceptors.

The expulsion rates are consistently lower for the high parity IUD acceptor than for the acceptor with a parity of 1 or 2.

Removal rates for bleeding or pain are also consistently lower among the high parity acceptor when compared to the acceptor with a parity of 1 or 2.

Taking parity as the distinguishing characteristic, and combining the risks of pregnancy, expulsion and removal, the high parity (3 and

continued overleaf

DEVICE	PREGNANCY	EXPULSION	REMOVAL FOR BLEEDING/PAIN
Gravigard (Copper 7)	LOW 1.6 ± 0.4	MODERATE 6.6 ± 0.9	MODERATE 8.9 ± 1.0
Gyne T (Copper T)	LOW 0.0	LOW 4.9 ± 1.5	MODERATE 6.0 ± 1.7
Antigon (Wing)	MODERATE 2.7 ± 1.5	MODERATE 6.6 ± 2.3	HIGH 10.4 ± 2.9

Based on one year of use. Figures represent net event rates (with S.E.) per 100 users, with at least 100 women remaining in the study during the twelfth month.

DEVICE INFORMATION	GENERAL CONSIDERATIONS
1. Average pregnancy, expulsion and removal rates. 2. Gradual increase in pregnancy rate, sharp decrease in expulsion rate and constant removal rate in second year of use. 3. Most accept another IUD after expulsion but not after a pregnancy or removal.	over) patient is clearly a more successful IUD user than the woman of lower parity. The difference is marked and applies to all the devices where a comparison can be made. The most appropriate devices for this group of patients are the Lippes Loop D, Gravigard and the Gyne T.
1. Lower than average pregnancy and removal rates; average expulsion rate. 2. Most accept another IUD after expulsion but not after a pregnancy or removal.	
1. Above average pregnancy rate; average expulsion and removal rates. 2. Most accept another IUD after expulsion but not after a pregnancy or removal.	

DEVICE	PREGNANCY	EXPULSION	REMOVAL FOR BLEEDING/PAIN
Lippes Loop B	LOW 1.2 ± 0.7	HIGH 11.7 ± 2.2	HIGH 11.3 ± 2.2
Lippes Loop C	LOW 1.6 ± 0.3	MODERATE 9.7 ± 0.7	HIGH 13.3 ± 0.8
Lippes Loop D	LOW 1.8 ± 0.4	MODERATE 6.3 ± 0.8	MODERATE 9.3 ± 1.0
Saf-T-Coil	LOW 1.8 ± 0.4	HIGH 11.2 ± 0.9	HIGH 13.3 ± 1.0

Based on one year of use. Figures represent net event rates (with S.E.) per 100 users, with at least 100 women remaining in the study during the twelfth month.

DEVICE INFORMATION	GENERAL CONSIDERATIONS
1. Average pregnancy, expulsion and removal rates. 2. Most accept another IUD after expulsion but not after pregnancy or removal.	*Pregnancy:* The pregnancy rates for this category of patient range from 0.6 to 2.7 per 100 users in the first year of IUD use and with most IUDs from 1.2 to 1.8. The exceptions are the Gyne T (Copper T) and the Wing Antigon, which show particularly low rates, and the Gravigard device which at 2.7 is the highest pregnancy rate recorded for these patients.
1. Average pregnancy, expulsion and removal rates. 2. Increase in pregnancy rate, sharp decrease in expulsion rate and gradual decrease in removal rate in second year of use. 3. Most accept another IUD after expulsion but not after a pregnancy or removal.	*Expulsion:* The Lippes Loop D shows the lowest and the Gravigard device the highest expulsion rates at one year of use with the majority of devices in the range of 9.7 to 11.7. *Removal:* The majority of devices have bleeding or pain removal rates in the range 9.3 to 13.3 per 100 users in one year. The Gyne T has a lower rate than this and the Film Antigon has an abnormally high removal rate at 17.4.
1. Average pregnancy rate; below average expulsion and removal rates. 2. Gradual decrease in pregnancy rate, sharp decrease in expulsion rate, and constant removal rate in second year of use. 3. Most accept another IUD after expulsion but not after a pregnancy or removal.	*Conclusion:* The pregnancy rates for these low age (under thirty years) patients are consistently but slightly higher than those for women aged thirty years and over. The one exception is the Wing Antigon. The expulsion rates are clearly and consistently higher among the lower age groups when compared to those aged thirty years and over. This difference is marked and relates to all devices where a comparison could be made.
1. Average pregnancy, expulsion and removal rates. 2. Gradual decrease in pregnancy, expulsion and removal rates in second year of use. 3. Most accept another IUD after expulsion but not after a pregnancy or removal.	A comparison of the removal rates between different age groups show no clear pattern. With some devices the removal rates are higher for the lower age group (e.g. Lippes Loop C, Wing Antigon) with other devices the lower age group exhibits lower removal rates (e.g. Lippes Loop D,

continued overleaf

DEVICE	PREGNANCY	EXPULSION	REMOVAL FOR BLEEDING/PAIN
Gravigard (Copper 7)	MODERATE 2.7 ± 0.2	HIGH 13.7 ± 0.5	MODERATE 9.4 ± 0.5
Gyne T (Copper T)	LOW 0.6 ± 0.4	MODERATE 7.4 ± 1.3	MODERATE 7.7 ± 1.3
Antigon (Wing)	LOW 0.8 ± 0.6	HIGH 10.7 ± 2.1	HIGH 13.1 ± 2.3
Antigon (Film)	LOW 1.4 ± 0.8	HIGH 10.5 ± 2.1	HIGH 17.4 ± 2.7

Based on one year of use. Figures represent net event rates (with S.E.) per 100 users, with at least 100 women remaining in the study during the twelfth month.

DEVICE INFORMATION	GENERAL CONSIDERATIONS
1. Above average pregnancy and expulsion rates; average removal rate. 2. Gradual decrease in pregnancy and removal rates and sharp decrease in expulsion rate in second year of use. 3. Most accept another IUD after expulsion but not after a pregnancy or removal.	Saf-T-Coil, Film Antigon). In the remainder, there appears to be little or no difference between the two groups (e.g. Gravigard and Gyne T). Taking age as the distinguishing characteristic, and combining the risks of pregnancy, expulsion and removal, the low age (under thirty years) patient is clearly a less successful IUD user than the older woman. The difference is marked and applies to all the devices where a comparison can be made. The most appropriate devices for this group of patients are the Lippes Loop C and the Lippes Loop D.
1. Below average pregnancy, expulsion and removal rates. 2. Gradual decrease in the pregnancy rate, sharp decrease in the expulsion rate and constant removal rate in second year of use. 3. Over 75 per cent accept another IUD after an expulsion but most refuse after a pregnancy or removal.	
1. Average pregnancy, expulsion and removal rates. 2. Constant pregnancy and removal rates and sharp decrease in expulsion rate in second year of use. 3. Over 75 per cent accept another IUD after expulsion but most refuse after a pregnancy or removal.	
1. Average pregnancy and expulsion rates; above average removal rate. 2. Most accept another IUD after expulsion but not after a pregnancy or removal.	

DEVICE	PREGNANCY	EXPULSION	REMOVAL FOR BLEEDING/PAIN
Lippes Loop C	LOW 0.7 ± 0.2	LOW 3.9 ± 0.6	HIGH 10.6 ± 1.0
Lippes Loop D	LOW 1.0 ± 0.4	LOW 3.7 ± 0.7	HIGH 11.2 ± 1.3
Saf-T-Coil (Standard)	LOW 0.8 ± 0.3	MODERATE 6.5 ± 0.8	HIGH 14.7 ± 1.2

Based on one year of use. Figures represent net event rates (with S.E.) per 100 users, with at least 100 women remaining in the study during the twelfth month.

DEVICE INFORMATION	GENERAL CONSIDERATIONS
1. Average pregnancy rate; below average expulsion and removal rates. 2. Constant pregnancy rate and gradual decrease in expulsion and removal rates in second year of use. 3. Over 75 per cent accept another IUD after expulsion but most refuse after a pregnancy or removal.	*Pregnancy:* The risk of pregnancy among these patients appears to be very low for all devices. This low risk may be reflecting the lower level of fecundity among these women. The IUD expulsion rates with this category of patient are also very low when compared to other age categories. The pregnancy rates range from nil (Gyne T) to 1.7 (Wing Antigon) with most devices in the range 0.6 to 1.0 per 100 users in the first year of use.
1. Average pregnancy and removal rates; lower than average expulsion rate. 2. Constant pregnancy rate and gradual decrease in expulsion and removal rates in second year of use. 3. Over 75 per cent accept another IUD after expulsion but most refuse after a pregnancy or removal.	*Expulsion:* The risk of expulsion is very low among these patients. With a range of between 3.3 and 6.5 in the first year of use, the rates obtained are the lowest for any group of patients differentiated by age or parity. *Removal:* The range of removal rates is very wide (7.7 to 19.9 per 100 users in the first year) with the majority of devices having rates between 9.5 and 11.2. The Gyne T (Copper T) has a lower rate of 7.7 and the Film Antigon a very high rate of 19.9. The standard size Saf-T-Coil also has a relatively high removal rate of 14.7.
1. Average pregnancy rate; above average expulsion and removal rates. 2. Sharp decrease in pregnancy and expulsion rates and gradual decrease in removal rate in second year of use. 3. Most accept another IUD after expulsion but not after a pregnancy or removal.	*Conclusion:* Patients in the higher age group of thirty years and over appear to be very suitable candidates for IUD use. In comparison with patients of lower age, the patient of thirty years and over is likely to experience a lower risk of pregnancy and IUD expulsion irrespective of the IUD model being worn. The removal rate is less consistent. With some devices the removal rate is lower (e.g. Lippes Loop C, Wing Antigon) with others higher (e.g. Lippes Loop D, Saf-T-Coil, Film Antigon) and in others about the same as *continued overleaf*

DEVICE	PREGNANCY	EXPULSION	REMOVAL FOR BLEEDING/PAIN
Gravigard (Copper 7)	LOW 0.6 ± 0.2	MODERATE 6.3 ± 0.6	MODERATE 9.5 ± 0.8
Gyne T (Copper T)	LOW 0.0	LOW 3.3 ± 1.0	MODERATE 7.7 ± 1.5
Antigon (Wing)	LOW 1.7 ± 1.1	MODERATE 6.3 ± 2.1	MODERATE 9.7 ± 2.6
Antigon (Film)	LOW 0.9 ± 0.8	MODERATE 5.6 ± 2.1	HIGH 19.9 ± 3.9

Based on one year of use. Figures represent net event rates (with S.E.) per 100 users, with at least 100 women remaining in the study during the twelfth month.

DEVICE INFORMATION	GENERAL CONSIDERATIONS
1. Average pregnancy and removal rates; above average expulsion rate. 2. Gradual decrease in pregnancy and removal rate and sharp decrease in expulsion rate in second year of use. 3. Most accept another IUD after expulsion but not after a pregnancy or removal.	those for younger women (e.g. Gravigard and Gyne T). When pregnancy, expulsion and removal rates are considered together, the higher age patient is clearly a more successful IUD user than the younger patient. The difference is marked and applies to all the devices where a comparison can be made. The most appropriate devices for these patients are the Lippes Loop C, the Lippes Loop D and the Gyne T.
1. Below average pregnancy, expulsion and removal rates. 2. Most accept another IUD after expulsion but not after a pregnancy or removal.	
1. Average pregnancy, expulsion and removal rates. 2. Most accept another IUD after expulsion but not after a pregnancy or removal.	
1. Average pregnancy and expulsion rates; above average removal rate. 2. Most accept another IUD after expulsion but not after a pregnancy or removal.	

DEVICE	PREGNANCY	EXPULSION	REMOVAL FOR BLEEDING/PAIN
Lippes Loop B	LOW 1.7 ± 1.0	HIGH 12.5 ± 2.7	HIGH 11.7 ± 2.6
Lippes Loop C	LOW 1.5 ± 0.3	HIGH 10.3 ± 0.8	HIGH 13.1 ± 0.9
Lippes Loop D	LOW 1.8 ± 0.5	MODERATE 6.5 ± 0.9	MODERATE 9.8 ± 1.1
Saf-T-Coil (Standard)	LOW 1.6 ± 0.4	HIGH 11.5 ± 1.0	HIGH 13.4 ± 1.1

Based on one year of use. Figures represent net event rates (with S.E.) per 100 users, with at least 100 women remaining in the study during the twelfth month.

DEVICE INFORMATION	GENERAL CONSIDERATIONS
1. Average pregnancy, expulsion and removal rates. 2. Most accept another IUD after expulsion but not after a pregnancy or removal.	*Pregnancy:* The risk of pregnancy among these patients ranges between 0.5 and 3.1 per 100 users during the first year of use depending on the IUD model being worn. Most of the rates lie in the narrower range 1.1 to 1.8. The exceptions are the Gyne T (Copper T) and the Wing Antigon which have lower rates and the Gravigard (Copper 7) which has a higher rate.
1. Average pregnancy, expulsion and removal rates. 2. Increase in pregnancy rate, sharp decrease in expulsion rate and constant removal rate in second year of use. 3. Most accept another IUD after expulsion but not after a pregnancy or removal.	*Expulsion:* The expulsion rates are all either moderate or high with a range of between 6.5 and 12.5 for every 100 users during the first year of use. The lowest rate is obtained with the Lippes Loop D and the highest with the Lippes Loop B. The copper carrying IUDs also show a wide range, with the Gyne T (Copper T) at 7.3 and the Gravigard (Copper 7) at 11.8 per 100 users.
1. Average pregnancy rate; below average expulsion and removal rates. 2. Gradual decrease in pregnancy rate, sharp decrease in expulsion rate and constant removal rate in second year of use. 3. Most accept another IUD after expulsion but not after a pregnancy or removal.	*Removal:* This category of patient shows high removal rates for most of the devices under review. The only exceptions are the Lippes Loop D and the Gyne T (Copper T) which have lower removal rates of 9.8 and 6.9 respectively.
1. Average pregnancy, expulsion and removal rates. 2. Gradual decrease in pregnancy, expulsion and removal rates in second year. 3. Most accept another IUD after expulsion but not after a pregnancy or removal.	*Conclusion:* The pregnancy rates with this category of patient are similar to those obtained with women of similar age but higher parity. The risk of pregnancy also appears to be higher than for older patients (thirty years and over) irrespective of their parity level. Age appears to be more important than parity levels in relation to the risk of pregnancy. The expulsion rates for this category of patient are consistently higher than those obtained for women of the same age but of higher parity. There exists a clear pattern in relation to expulsion

continued overleaf

DEVICE	PREGNANCY	EXPULSION	REMOVAL FOR BLEEDING/PAIN
Gravigard (Copper 7)	MODERATE 3.1 ± 0.4	HIGH 11.8 ± 0.8	HIGH 10.0 ± 0.7
Gyne T (Copper T)	LOW 0.7 ± 0.5	MODERATE 7.3 ± 1.5	MODERATE 6.9 ± 1.5
Antigon (Wing)	LOW 0.5 ± 0.5	HIGH 11.9 ± 2.5	HIGH 13.4 ± 2.6
Antigon (Film)	LOW 1.1 ± 0.8	HIGH 11.9 ± 2.5	HIGH 18.7 ± 3.1

Based on one year of use. Figures represent net event rates (with S.E.) per 100 users, with at least 100 women remaining in the study during the twelfth month.

DEVICE INFORMATION	GENERAL CONSIDERATIONS
1. Above average pregnancy rate; average expulsion and removal rates. 2. Gradual decrease in pregnancy and removal rates and sharp decrease in expulsion rate in second year of use. 3. Over 75 per cent accept another IUD after expulsion but most refuse after a pregnancy or removal.	rates depending on the age and parity of the IUD acceptor. The low age, low parity (1 or 2) patient produces the highest expulsion rates followed by those of low age and high parity and then by those of high age and low parity. The lowest expulsion rates are found among those patients over thirty years of age with a parity of 3 or more.
1. Below average pregnancy, expulsion and removal rates. 2. Most accept another IUD after an expulsion but not after a pregnancy or removal.	When compared with other age and parity categories removal for bleeding or pain does not show a consistent pattern. Age and parity do not appear to be the determining factors in the rate of IUD removals following a complaint of bleeding or pain. The most appropriate devices for these patients are the Lippes Loop D and the Gyne T.
1. Below average pregnancy rate; average expulsion rate; above average removal rate. 2. Over 75 per cent accept another IUD after expulsion but most refuse after a pregnancy or removal.	
1. Average pregnancy and expulsion rates; above average removal rate. 2. Over 75 per cent accept another IUD after expulsion but most refuse after a pregnancy or removal.	

DEVICE	PREGNANCY	EXPULSION	REMOVAL FOR BLEEDING/PAIN
Lippes Loop C	LOW 1.5 ± 0.7	MODERATE 5.9 ± 1.4	HIGH 14.4 ± 2.2
Lippes Loop D	LOW 1.7 ± 0.9	MODERATE 5.1 ± 1.6	MODERATE 5.9 ± 1.7
Saf-T-Coil (Standard)	LOW 1.8 ± 0.9	MODERATE 8.8 ± 1.9	HIGH 13.6 ± 2.4
Gravigard (Copper 7)	MODERATE 4.4 ± 1.2	MODERATE 8.7 ± 1.7	MODERATE 9.7 ± 1.8

Based on one year of use. Figures represent net event rates (with S.E.) per 100 users, with at least 100 women remaining in the study during the twelfth month.

DEVICE INFORMATION	GENERAL CONSIDERATIONS
1. Average pregnancy and expulsion rates; above average removal rate. 2. Most accept another IUD after expulsion but not after a pregnancy or removal.	*Pregnancy:* The pregnancy rates for this category of patient are similar to those obtained among women of similar age but lower parity. The risk of pregnancy also appears to be higher than that obtained among older women (thirty years and over) irrespective of their parity level. Age appears to be more important than parity in relation to the risk of pregnancy.
1. Average pregnancy rate; below average expulsion and removal rates. 2. Over 75 per cent accept another IUD after expulsion but most refuse after a pregnancy or removal.	*Expulsion:* The expulsion rates for this category of patient are consistently lower than those obtained for women of the same age but of lower parity. There is a clear pattern in relation to expulsion rates depending on the age and parity of the IUD acceptor. The highest expulsion rates are found among the low age (under thirty years), low parity (1 or 2) IUD acceptor. These are followed by the low age, high parity (3 or over) acceptor and the high age, low parity acceptor. The lowest expulsion rates are found among those patients over thirty years of age with a parity of 3 or more.
1. Average pregnancy and expulsion rates; above average removal rate. 2. Most accept another IUD after an expulsion but not after a pregnancy or removal.	*Removal:* When compared with other age and parity categories, removal for bleeding or pain does not show a consistent pattern. Age and parity do not appear to be the determining factors in the rate of IUD removal following a complaint of bleeding or pain.
1. Above average pregnancy and expulsion rates; average removal rate. 2. Most accept another IUD after an expulsion but not after a pregnancy or removal.	*Conclusion:* The most appropriate devices for these patients is the Lippes Loop D.

DEVICE	PREGNANCY	EXPULSION	REMOVAL FOR BLEEDING/PAIN
Lippes Loop C	LOW 0.6 ± 0.3	LOW 4.7 ± 0.8	HIGH 12.1 ± 1.3
Lippes Loop D	LOW 1.1 ± 0.6	LOW 3.5 ± 1.0	HIGH 11.8 ± 1.9
Saf-T-Coil (Standard)	LOW 0.6 ± 0.3	MODERATE 8.5 ± 1.3	HIGH 15.9 ± 1.7
Gravigard (Copper 7)	LOW 0.8 ± 0.3	MODERATE 5.9 ± 0.8	HIGH 11.0 ± 1.1
Gyne T (Copper T)	LOW 0.0	LOW 2.3 ± 1.1	MODERATE 9.9 ± 2.3

Based on one year of use. Figures represent net event rates (with S.E.) per 100 users, with at least 100 women remaining in the study during the twelfth month.

DEVICE INFORMATION	GENERAL CONSIDERATIONS
1. Average pregnancy, expulsion and removal rates. 2. Constant pregnancy rate and gradually decreasing expulsion and removal rates in the second year of use. 3. Most accept another IUD after expulsion but not after a pregnancy or removal.	*Pregnancy:* The pregnancy rates for this category of patient are similar to those obtained among women of similar age but higher parity. The risk of pregnancy is also lower than that obtained among younger women (under thirty years) irrespective of their parity level. Age appears to be more important than parity levels in relation to the risk of pregnancy.
1. Average pregnancy, expulsion and removal rates. 2. Sharp decrease in the pregnancy rate, gradual decrease in the expulsion rate and constant removal rate in the second year of use. 3. Most accept another IUD after expulsion but not after a pregnancy or removal.	*Expulsion:* There is a clear pattern in relation to expulsion rates depending on the age and parity of the IUD acceptor. The highest expulsion rates are found among the low age, low parity patients. These are followed by the low age, high parity acceptor and the high age, low parity acceptor. The lowest expulsion rates are found among those patients over thirty years of age with a parity of 3 or more.
1. Average pregnancy rate; above average expulsion and removal rates. 2. Sharp decrease in pregnancy and expulsion rates, and gradual decrease in the removal rate in the second year of use. 3. Most accept another IUD after expulsion but not after a pregnancy or removal.	*Removal:* When compared with other age and parity categories, removal for bleeding or pain does not show a consistent pattern. Age and parity do not appear to be determining factors in the rate of IUD removal following a complaint of bleeding or pain.
1. Average pregnancy, expulsion and removal rates. 2. Gradual decrease in pregnancy and removal rates and sharp decrease in expulsion rate in second year of use. 3. Most accept another IUD after expulsion but not after a pregnancy or removal.	*Conclusion:* The most appropriate devices for these patients are the Lippes Loop C, Lippes Loop D and the Gyne T.
1. Below average pregnancy, expulsion and removal rates. 2. Over 75 per cent accept another IUD after expulsion but most refuse after a pregnancy or removal.	

DEVICE	PREGNANCY	EXPULSION	REMOVAL FOR BLEEDING/PAIN
Lippes Loop C	LOW 0.8 ± 0.4	LOW 2.9 ± 0.8	MODERATE 8.0 ± 1.3
Lippes Loop D	LOW 0.9 ± 0.5	LOW 4.0 ± 1.1	HIGH 10.8 ± 1.7
Saf-T-Coil (Standard)	LOW 0.9 ± 0.5	LOW 4.0 ± 1.0	HIGH 13.2 ± 1.8

Based on one year of use. Figures represent net event rates (with S.E.) per 100 users, with at least 100 women remaining in the study during the twelfth month.

DEVICE INFORMATION	GENERAL CONSIDERATIONS
1. Average pregnancy and removal rates; below average expulsion rate. 2. Gradual decrease in pregnancy and expulsion rates and constant removal rate in second year of use. 3. Over 75 per cent accept another IUD after expulsion but most refuse after a pregnancy or removal.	*Pregnancy:* The pregnancy rates for this category of patient are similar to those obtained among women of similar age but lower parity. The risk of pregnancy is also lower than that found among younger women irrespective of their parity level. Age appears to be more important than parity levels in relation to the risk of pregnancy.
1. Average pregnancy, expulsion and removal rates. 2. Increase in pregnancy rate, sharp decrease in expulsion rate and constant removal rate in second year of use. 3. Over 75 per cent accept another IUD after expulsion but most refuse after a pregnancy or removal.	*Expulsion:* There is a clear pattern in relation to expulsion rates depending on the age and parity of the IUD acceptor. The highest expulsion rates are found among the low age, low parity patients. These are followed by the low age, high parity acceptor and the high age, low parity acceptor. The lowest expulsion rates are found among those patients over thirty years of age with a parity of 3 or more. *Removal:* No consistent pattern emerges across age and parity groups in relation to IUD removal. Age and parity do not appear to be determining factors in the rate of IUD removal following a complaint of bleeding or pain.
1. Average pregnancy and expulsion rates; above average removal rate. 2. Sharp decrease in pregnancy and expulsion rates and gradual decrease in removal rate in second year of use. 3. Most accept another IUD after expulsion but not after a pregnancy or removal.	*Conclusion:* The most appropriate device for these patients is the Lippes Loop C.

PART 2: THE IUD MODEL

This part of Section II contains data relating to the following IUDs:

1. Lippes Loop B
2. Lippes Loop C
3. Lippes Loop D
4. Saf-T-Coil 33S
5. Gravigard (Copper 7)
6. Gyne T (Copper T)
7. Wing Antigon
8. Film Antigon

IUD s not commonly fitted at the present time are also described:

Copper Omega
Dalkon Shield
Multiload
Progestasert

GENERAL INFORMATION

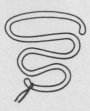

Composition: Polyethylene impregnated with barium sulphate to permit X-ray visualisation. Monofilament tail: 2 black threads.

Size: Overall length 27.5 mm. Width at widest point 27.5 mm.

Surface area: 781 mm²

Inserter size: 5.0 mm × 4.0 mm outside diameter (rectangular shape with rounded edges).

Usual method of insertion: Push technique.

Duration of use: Indefinite.

Use: Limited use in the United Kingdom when compared to the larger sizes of Lippes Loop (2.2 per cent of all first fittings in the IUD network between 1972 and 1976.

Pelvic Inflammatory Disease: One reported case for every 385 women wearing the device for one year. This is the lowest rate recorded for all devices in general use at the present time.

Perforation: No uterine or cervical perforations were reported with this device. (422 fittings.)

Unwanted pregnancy outcome: Of those wishing to continue with the pregnancy abour 50 per cent have a successful confinement.

GENERAL COMMENT

The pregnancy rates for this device are as low as those obtained for all other devices with the exception of the Gyne T (Copper T), which has a lower pregnancy rate.

The expulsion rates at the end of the first year of use are similar to those for the Saf-T-Coil and Antigon devices; and consistently higher than those for the Lippes Loop sizes C and D and the Gyne T. A comparison with the Gravigard indicates that there are no consistent differences in the expulsion rates. For some age and parity groups the rate is higher among Lippes Loop B users but in other groups the reverse is demonstrated.

The bleeding/pain removal rates are lower than those for the Saf-T-Coil, Lippes Loop C and the Antigon devices; similar to those for the Lippes Loop D, the Gravigard (Copper 7) and higher than those for the Gyne T (Copper T).

Owing to the small number of fittings with this device (2.2 per cent of total) it is not possible for us to calculate rates beyond twelve months of use. It is intriguing that this device is not more popular than it appears. Inflammatory complications are rare; there are no perforations reported; the pregnancy rate is comparable to other devices and the bleeding/pain removals are lower than those reported for the more popular Lippes Loop C. The device does have consistently higher expulsion rates than most other IUDs in current use, but the differences are not marked.

Supplier: Ortho Pharmaceutical Ltd.

	PREGNANCY	EXPULSION	REMOVAL FOR BLEEDING/PAIN
All First Fittings	LOW 1.1 ± 0.6	MODERATE 9.2 ± 1.6	HIGH 11.0 ± 1.8
All Parous	LOW 1.3 ± 0.7	MODERATE 8.5 ± 1.7	MODERATE 9.7 ± 1.8
Parity 1 & 2	LOW 1.7 ± 0.8	HIGH 10.6 ± 2.1	.HIGH 10.2 ± 2.1
Age — Under 30	LOW 1.2 ± 0.7	HIGH 11.7 ± 2.2	HIGH 11.3 ± 2.2
Under 30 Parity 1 & 2	LOW 1.7 ± 1.0	HIGH 12.5 ± 2.7	HIGH 11.7 ± 2.6

Based on one year of use. Figures represent net event rates (with S.E.) per 100 users with at least 100 women remaining in the study during the twelfth month.

GENERAL INFORMATION	GENERAL COMMENT

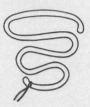

Composition: Polyethylene impregnated with barium sulphate to permit X-ray visualisation. Monofilament tail: 2 yellow threads.

Size: Overall length 30.0 mm. Width at widest point 30.95 mm.

Surface area: 920 mm^2.

Inserter size: 5.0 mm × 4.0 mm outside measurement. (Rectangular shape with rounded edges.)

Usual method of insertion: Push technique.

Duration of use: Indefinite.

Use: Second most commonly fitted IUD in the United Kingdom (19.2 per cent of all IUD first fittings among the clinics in the IUD network).

Pelvic Inflammatory Disease: A total of 21 cases were reported, one case for every 195 Lippes Loop C users for each year of use. Just over half this total had the IUD removed during treatment.

Perforation: There were 1.2 uterine perforations for evert 1,000 fittings. No cervical perforations have been reported.

Unwanted pregnancy outcome: Of those wishing to continue with the pregnancy just over half had a successful confinement.

This very popular device has a consistently low pregnancy rate which tends to decrease with each year of continued use. The pregnancy rate for the second year is similar to that for the first year but there is a decrease in the third year. This pregnancy rate is consistent with the rates obtained for all other devices with the exception of copper carrying IUDs. The Lippes Loop C has a higher pregnancy rate than the Gyne T but a lower pregnancy rate than the Gravigard in most age and parity categories of IUD user.

The expulsion rate is slightly higher than that obtained with the Lippes Loop D and the Gyne T but lower than that obtained with all other devices fitted in the clinic network between 1972 and 1976. This comparatively low expulsion rate tends to decrease over the first three years of use — over 50 per cent of all expulsions occur within three months of fitting. Most patients who experience an expulsion of the device are refitted with another IUD.

The removal rate following complaints of bleeding and/or pain is similar to that obtained with the Saf-T-Coil (except in the high age group when the rate for the Lippes Loop C is lower), and the Wing Antigon but higher than for the Lippes Loop D, B, Gravigard and Gyne T. The Film Antigon is the only device which has a higher bleeding/pain removal rate in all age and parity categories of patient. There is a gradual decrease in the Lippes Loop C removal rate over the first three years of use.

This device is available by prescription within the National Health Service (United Kingdom).

Supplier: Ortho Pharmaceutical Ltd.

	PREGNANCY	EXPULSION	REMOVAL FOR BLEEDING/PAIN
All First Fittings	LOW 1.2 ± 0.2	MODERATE 7.4 ± 0.5	HIGH 12.3 ± 0.6
All Parous	LOW 1.2 ± 0.2	MODERATE 7.3 ± 0.5	HIGH 12.2 ± 0.6
Parity 1 & 2	LOW 1.2 ± 0.2	MODERATE 8.5 ± 0.6	HIGH 12.9 ± 0.8
Parity 3 or More	LOW 1.2 ± 0.4	LOW 4.0 ± 0.7	HIGH 10.4 ± 1.2
Age — Under 30	LOW 1.6 ± 0.3	MODERATE 9.7 ± 0.7	HIGH 13.3 ± 0.8
Age — 30 & Over	LOW 0.7 ± 0.2	LOW 3.9 ± 0.6	HIGH 10.6 ± 1.0
Under 30 Parity 1 & 2	LOW 1.5 ± 0.3	HIGH 10.3 ± 0.8	HIGH 13.1 ± 0.9
Under 30 Parity 3 or More	LOW 1.5 ± 0.7	MODERATE 5.9 ± 1.4	HIGH 14.4 ± 2.2
30 & Over Parity 1 & 2	LOW 0.6 ± 0.3	LOW 4.7 ± 0.8	HIGH 12.1 ± 1.3
30 & Over Parity 3 or More	LOW 0.8 ± 0.4	LOW 2.9 ± 0.8	MODERATE 8.0 ± 1.3

ed on one year of use. Figures represent net event rates (with S.E.) per 100 users with at least 100 women remaining in study during the twelfth month.

GENERAL INFORMATION

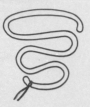

Composition: Polyethylene impregnated with barium suphate to permit X-ray visualisation. Monofilament tail: 2 white threads.

Size: Overall length 30.0 mm. Width at widest point 30.0 mm. The plastic rod from which Loop D is made is thicker and more rigid than that used for Loop C.

Surface area: 951 mm^2.

Inserter size: 5.0 mm × 4.0 mm outside measurement. (Rectangular shape with rounded edges.)

Usual method of insertion: Push technique.

Duration of use: Indefinite.

Use: Frequently fitted in the United Kingdom. (10 per cent of fittings among the clinics in the IUD network.)

Pelvic Inflammatory Disease: A total of seven cases were reported which yields one case for every 342 Lippes Loop D users for each year of use. This rate is the second lowest rate for inflammatory disease reported in the IUD network.

Perforation: There were 3.4 perforations for every 1,000 fittings. No cervical perforations have been reported.

Unwanted pregnancy outcome: Of those wishing to continue with the pregnancy just over two thirds had a successful confinement.

GENERAL COMMENT

The pregnancy rates obtained with this device are as low as those obtained with the other Lippes Loop devices, Saf-T-Coil and the Antigon models. These rates are generally higher than those obtained for the Gyne T and lower than those obtained for the Gravigard. There is evidence of a gradual decrease in the pregnancy rates over the first three years of use with the Lippes Loop D.

The expulsion rates are generally lower than those for the Lippes Loop C with the exception of the high parity acceptor category. The rates of expulsion are also lower than those for the Saf-T-Coil, Antigon and Gravigard devices. The only comparably low expulsion rates are those associated with the use of the Gyne T. The rates decrease very sharply with increasing duration of use, most expulsions occurring during the first three months. Expulsion rates for the second and third years of use are only a fraction of those obtained in the first year.

The Lippes Loop D demonstrates the lowest rate of bleeding/pain removal of all the non-copper devices being fitted in the IUD network of clinics. The rates are comparable to those obtained with the Gravigard but slightly greater than those obtained with the Gyne T. The rate of removal at the end of the first year remains fairly constant over the following two years.

Most users experiencing an expulsion of the device are refitted with another IUD but those experiencing a pregnancy or a removal for bleeding or pain generally refuse another IUD.

This device is available by prescription within the National Health Service (United Kingdom).

Supplier: Ortho Pharmaceutical Ltd.

	PREGNANCY	EXPULSION	REMOVAL FOR BLEEDING/PAIN
All First Fittings	LOW 1.4 ± 0.3	MODERATE 5.2 ± 0.6	HIGH 10.1 ± 0.8
All Parous	LOW 1.5 ± 0.3	MODERATE 5.1 ± 0.6	HIGH 10.0 ± 0.8
Parity 1 & 2	LOW 1.6 ± 0.4	MODERATE 5.5 ± 0.7	HIGH 10.4 ± 1.0
Parity 3 or More	LOW 1.2 ± 0.5	LOW 4.4 ± 0.9	MODERATE 9.0 ± 1.3
Age — Under 30	LOW 1.8 ± 0.4	MODERATE 6.3 ± 0.8	MODERATE 9.3 ± 1.0
Age — 30 & Over	LOW 1.0 ± 0.4	LOW 3.7 ± 0.7	HIGH 11.2 ± 1.3
Under 30 **Parity 1 & 2**	LOW 1.8 ± 0.5	MODERATE 6.5 ± 0.9	MODERATE 9.8 ± 1.1
Under 30 **Parity 3 or More**	LOW 1.7 ± 0.9	MODERATE 5.1 ± 1.6	MODERATE 5.9 ± 1.7
30 & Over **Parity 1 & 2**	LOW 1.1 ± 0.6	LOW 3.5 ± 1.0	HIGH 11.8 ± 1.9
30 & Over **Parity 3 or More**	LOW 0.9 ± 0.5	LOW 4.0 ± 1.1	HIGH 10.8 ± 1.7

Based on one year of use. Figures represent net event rates (with S.E.) per 100 users with at least 100 women remaining in the study during the twelfth month.

GENERAL INFORMATION	GENERAL COMMENT

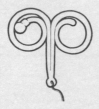

Composition: Polyethylene impregnated with barium sulphate to permit X-ray visualisation.

Size (33SX): Overall length 30.7 – 34.3 mm. Width at widest point 36.8 – 39.4 mm.

Surface area: 1,064 mm^2.

Inserter size: Outside diameter: 4.45 – 4.57 mm.

Usual method of insertion: Pull back outer sleeve of inserter.

Duration of use: Indefinite.

Use: An IUD which has been fitted in the United Kingdom for about ten years. Represents 14.4 per cent of all IUD first fittings reported in the IUD network.

Pelvic Inflammatory Disease: One reported case for every 274 Saf-T-Coil users per year indicates that this device is as safe as the Lippes Loop devices and the Gyne T.

Perforation: No cases of perforation have been reported for this device in the IUD clinic network during the period of observation (1972–1976) involving 2,737 fittings.

Unwanted pregnancy outcome: Of the thirty-five cases where outcome of pregnancy is known, most were ended by a therapeutic abortion. Of the remainder, over two thirds resulted in a successful confinement; a third had a spontaneous abortion.

This device is associated with a pregnancy rate of between 0.8 and 1.8 per 100 users during the first year of use. This is a low rate and is comparable to the other non-copper carrying IUDs such as the Lippes Loop and the Antigon devices. The pregnancy rate is also consistently lower than that obtained with the Gravigard device but higher than that for the Gyne T.

The expulsion rate tends to be higher in all categories when compared to the Lippes Loop D, Lippes Loop C and the Antigon devices. The device also has higher expulsion rates than those obtained for the Gyne T but has comparable rates to the Gravigard device. It should be noted that there is a decrease in the expulsion rate over time but for most categories of women this decrease is gradual and does not exhibit the rapid decline demonstrated with many other devices over the first few months of use.

The Saf-T-Coil is removed for bleeding and/or pain at a higher rate than any other device with the exception of the Film Antigon. This finding holds with all categories of age and parity.

This device is available by prescription within the National Health Service (United Kingdom) at the present time.

Supplier: LR Industries Ltd.

	PREGNANCY	EXPULSION	REMOVAL FOR BLEEDING/PAIN
All First Fittings	LOW 1.4 ± 0.2	MODERATE 9.3 ± 0.6	HIGH 13.9 ± 0.8
All Parous	LOW 1.2 ± 0.2	MODERATE 9.2 ± 0.6	HIGH 13.9 ± 0.8
Parity 1 & 2	LOW 1.3 ± 0.3	HIGH 10.5 ± 0.8	HIGH 14.2 ± 0.9
Parity 3 or More	LOW 1.2 ± 0.4	MODERATE 6.0 ± 1.0	HIGH 13.3 ± 1.4
Age — Under 30	LOW 1.8 ± 0.4	HIGH 11.2 ± 0.9	HIGH 13.3 ± 1.0
Age -- 30 & Over	LOW 0.8 ± 0.3	MODERATE 6.5 ± 0.8	HIGH 14.7 ± 1.2
Under 30 Parity 1 & 2	LOW 1.6 ± 0.4	HIGH 11.5 ± 1.0	HIGH 13.4 ± 1.1
Under 30 Parity 3 or More	LOW 1.8 ± 0.9	MODERATE 8.8 ± 1.9	HIGH 13.6 ± 2.4
30 & Over Parity 1 & 2	LOW 0.6 ± 0.3	MODERATE 8.5 ± 1.3	HIGH 15.9 ± 1.7
30 & Over Parity 3 or More	LOW 0.9 ± 0.5	LOW 4.0 ± 1.0	HIGH 13.2 ± 1.8

ased on one year of use. Figures represent net event rates (with S.E.) per 100 users with at least 100 women remaining in he study during the twelfth month.

GENERAL INFORMATION

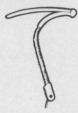

Composition: Polypropylene carrier impregnated with barium sulphate and carrying 89 mg of copper.

Size: Overall length 35.9 mm. Width at widest point 26 mm.

Surface area: Total surface area 330 mm² including 200 mm² of copper.

Inserter size: Outside diameter 3.0 mm.

Usual method of insertion: Either push or pull technique.

Duration of use: Two years — but see comments below.

Use: Frequently fitted in the United Kingdom (40.9 per cent of all first fittings reported by clinics in the IUD network).

Pelvic Inflammatory Disease: The incidence of one case in every 104 Gravigard acceptors per year is comparatively high compared to other IUD models. This is the highest rate reported in the IUD network and may be a result of the lower age and parity of those accepting this device.

Perforation: Five cases of perforation have been reported giving a rate of 0.6 cases in every 1,000 Gravigard fittings. Two of these were cervical perforations.

Unwanted pregnancy outcome: About half of all women becoming pregnant had the pregnancy terminated by therapeutic abortion. Of the remainder (those wishing to continue with pregnancy) just over half of the pregnancies ended in a successful confinement.

GENERAL COMMENT

This device is reported as being very easy to fit and the very low perforation rate appears to support this. Some doctors prefer to use a Copper 7 in their nulliparous patients owing to the ease of fitting (and see the rates given for the nulliparous patient on p. 52). One disadvantage is that the pregnancy rate with this device is somewhat higher than that obtained for most other devices in current use. The higher pregnancy rate is most obvious for those under thirty years of age, irrespective of parity.

The expulsion rate is also higher with this device with all categories of user, when compared to the other IUD models described in this manual. It would appear from these data that expulsion of the device is related to the pregnancy rate.

Removal for bleeding and/or pain tends to be lower with this device than with most other devices.

Among nulliparous patients the pregnancy rate remains constant over the first three years of use but among parous women the annual pregnancy rate is seen to gradually decrease. The expected rise in the pregnancy rate during the third year of use was not found. As with other devices there is a sharp decrease in the expulsion rate with years of use and a gradual decrease in the bleeding/pain removal rate.

This device is available by prescription within the National Health Service (United Kingdom).

Supplier: G.D. Searle and Co Ltd.

	PREGNANCY	EXPULSION	REMOVAL FOR BLEEDING/PAIN
All First Fittings	MODERATE 2.1 ± 0.2	HIGH 11.7 ± 0.4	MODERATE 9.4 ± 0.4
Nulliparous	MODERATE 2.0 ± 0.3	HIGH 15.3 ± 0.8	MODERATE 8.5 ± 0.6
All Parous	MODERATE 2.2 ± 0.2	MODERATE 9.1 ± 0.5	HIGH 10.0 ± 0.5
Parity 1 & 2	MODERATE 2.3 ± 0.3	MODERATE 9.9 ± 0.6	HIGH 10.3 ± 0.6
Parity 3 or More	LOW 1.6 ± 0.4	MODERATE 6.6 ± 0.9	MODERATE 8.9 ± 1.0
Age — Under 30	MODERATE 2.7 ± 0.2	HIGH 13.7 ± 0.5	MODERATE 9.4 ± 0.5
Age — 30 & Over	LOW 0.6 ± 0.2	MODERATE 6.3 ± 0.6	MODERATE 9.5 ± 0.8
Under 30 Parity 1 & 2	MODERATE 3.1 ± 0.4	HIGH 11.8 ± 0.8	HIGH 10.0 ± 0.7
Under 30 Parity 3 or More	MODERATE 4.4 ± 1.2	MODERATE 8.7 ± 1.7	MODERATE 9.7 ± 1.8
30 & Over Parity 1 & 2	LOW 0.8 ± 0.3	MODERATE 5.9 ± 0.8	HIGH 11.0 ± 1.1

ased on one year of use. Figures represent net event rates (with S.E.) per 100 users with at least 100 women remaining in
e study during the twelfth month.

GENERAL INFORMATION

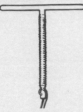

Composition: Polyethylene carrier supporting 120 mg of 0.25 mm diameter copper wire.

Size: Overall length (vertical) 38 mm. Width at widest point (horizontal) 32 mm.

Surface area: Total surface area 376 mm^2 including 200 mm^2 of copper.

Inserter size: Outside diameter 2.0 mm.

Usual method of insertion: Pull back outer inserter sleeve.

Duration of use: Two years.

Use: A relatively new device which is being fitted in large numbers in the United Kingdom (7.7 per cent of all first fittings reported in the IUD network).

Pelvic Inflammatory Disease: The rate of one reported case for every 253 Gyne T users per year is slightly more than average for all the IUDs being compared. Three of the four reported cases were treated without removal of the IUD.

Perforation: Only one case of perforation has been reported giving a crude rate of 0.7 per 1,000 fittings. This is a very low rate.

Unwanted pregnancy outcome: Only four pregnancies have been reported among women using this device in the period covered in this survey. Two of these pregnancies ended in a successful confinement; two ended in apparently spontaneous abortion.

GENERAL COMMENT

Like the Gravigard device, the Gyne T has a very low rate of perforation. This low rate appears to be related to the inserter size and the consequent ease of insertion rather than to the overall size of the device. This reinforces the view that the perforation of an IUD is relating to problems with fitting.

Where expulsion and removal rates can be given, these appear to be very low when compared to those for the traditional devices such as the Lippes Loop and the Saf-T-Coil and lower than those for the Gravigard device.

Event rates have been obtained for two years of use and the pregnancy rate, unlike that with other devices, has tended to increase with continued use. The expulsion rate drops in the second year of use but the rate of decrease is not as rapid as that obtained with other devices. There is a gradual decrease in removals for bleeding and pain.

The data collected in the IUD network indicates that this device is successful during the first year of use. The disadvantages at the present time are that it is said to require replacement at the end of two years and that it is *not* available by prescription within the National Health Service (United Kingdom). It is a relatively new device and it is known that reported rates tend to be lower during the first year or two following the introduction of a new device. For this reason, care should be exercised in interpreting the data presented.

Supplier: Ortho Pharmaceutical Ltd.

	PREGNANCY	EXPULSION	REMOVAL FOR BLEEDING/PAIN
All First Fittings	LOW 0.4 ± 0.2	MODERATE 5.7 ± 0.8	MODERATE 7.6 ± 1.0
All Parous	LOW 0.3 ± 0.2	MODERATE 5.2 ± 0.9	MODERATE 7.4 ± 1.0
Parity 1 & 2	LOW 0.5 ± 0.3	MODERATE 5.3 ± 1.0	MODERATE 8.1 ± 1.3
Parity 3 or More	LOW 0.0	LOW 4.9 ± 1.5	MODERATE 6.0 ± 1.7
Age — Under 30	LOW 0.6 ± 0.4	MODERATE 7.4 ± 1.3	MODERATE 7.7 ± 1.3
Age — 30 & Over	LOW 0.0	LOW 3.3 ± 1.0	MODERATE 7.7 ± 1.5
Under 30 Parity 1 & 2	LOW 0.7 ± 0.5	MODERATE 7.3 ± 1.5	MODERATE 6.9 ± 1.5
30 & Over Parity 1 & 2	LOW 0.0	LOW 2.3 ± 1.1	MODERATE 9.9 ± 2.3

sed on one year of use. Figures represent net event rates (with S.E.) per 100 users with at least 100 women remaining in
study during the twelfth month.

GENERAL INFORMATION

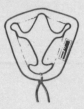

Composition: Polyethylene: fitted with small magnet for device detection.

Size: Overall length 27.5 mm. Width at widest point 26 mm.

Surface area: 1,057 mm^2.

Inserter size: The inserter does not have to pass into the cervical canal.

Usual method of insertion: The device is placed in the inserter. The head of the folded device is then placed against the external os of the cervix. The device is then pushed out of the inserter and thrust through the cervical canal by means of a plunger.

Duration of use: Indefinite.

Use: This device has been available for some years and is often used by doctors for patients who experience expulsion with other devices. This report is concerned only with first fittings of the device which represents 2.2 per cent of all first fittings reported in the IUD network during the period 1972–6.

Pelvic Inflammatory Disease: Five cases have been reported giving a crude rate of one case for every 125 Antigon users per year of observation. This is a high rate when compared to other devices.

Perforation: No cases of perforation of the uterus with this device were reported during the period of observation involving 421 fittings.

Unwanted pregnancy outcome: As with other devices most patients apply for and are given a therapeutic abortion but among the twenty pregnancies where the pregnancy continued slightly more ended in apparently spontaneous abortions than in a successful confinement.

GENERAL COMMENT

Many doctors claim that the Antigon is difficult to fit but once fitted the device is a satisfactory one. The data supports the view that there is a low pregnancy rate; the expulsion and removal rates are average when compared to other devices. The device is comparable to the Saf-T-Coil and clearly superior to the Film Antigon in relation to the rate of bleeding/pain removal.

There is a sharp decrease in the pregnancy and expulsion rates when comparing the first and second years of use but the removal rate for bleeding and pain remains relatively constant. (See also p. 100 for a description of the Film Antigon.)

This device is *not* available by prescription within the National Health Service (United Kingdom) at the present time.

Supplier: Svend Schroder.

	PREGNANCY	EXPULSION	REMOVAL FOR BLEEDING/PAIN
All First Fittings	LOW 1.1 ± 0.5	MODERATE 9.0 ± 1.5	HIGH 11.8 ± 1.8
All Parous	LOW 1.1 ± 0.5	MODERATE 9.1 ± 1.5	HIGH 11.9 ± 1.8
Parity 1 & 2	LOW 0.4 ± 0.4	HIGH 10.2 ± 2.0	HIGH 12.6 ± 2.2
Parity 3 or More	MODERATE 2.7 ± 1.5	MODERATE 6.6 ± 2.3	HIGH 10.4 ± 2.9
Age — Under 30	LOW 0.8 ± 0.6	HIGH 10.7 ± 2.1	HIGH 13.1 ± 2.3
Age — 30 & Over	LOW 1.7 ± 1.1	MODERATE 6.3 ± 2.1	MODERATE 9.7 ± 2.6
Under 30 Parity 1 & 2	LOW 0.5 ± 0.5	HIGH 11.9 ± 2.5	HIGH 13.4 ± 2.6

sed on one year of use. Figures represent net event rates (with S.E.) per 100 users with at least 100 women remaining in study during the twelfth month.

GENERAL INFORMATION

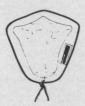

This device is very similar to the Wing Antigon
in terms of composition, insertion technique and
duration of use but has a larger surface area
(1,725 mm^2). The central area of the device is
covered with a thin layer of plastic and this is in
contrast to the 'Wing' model which only partly
encloses this central area. The prototype of the
Antigon device has neither 'wings' nor 'film'
but in other respects is similar to the later models.
It was believed that by presenting a larger surface
area to the endometrium, the pregnancy rate
would be lower without this change in design
affecting the expulsion and removal rates.

Use: The number of fittings is relatively small
(2.1 per cent of the total) but sufficient data has
been collected to suggest that the early claims for
this device have not been realised. Both the
pregnancy and expulsion rates are similar to those
obtained with other devices but the removal rate
is very high. This device conveys the highest rate
of removal for bleeding or pain for any device
considered in recent years. On average,
approximately 18 per cent of all acceptors have
had the device removed by the end of the first
year of use. This rises to a cumulative total of 35
per cent by the end of the second year. The larger
surface area in contact with the endometrium
does not appear to affect the pregnancy or
expulsion rates and the removal rate for bleeding

or pain appears to be high.

This device is *not* available by prescription within
the National Health Service (United Kingdom)
at the present time.

Supplier: Svend Schroder.

	PREGNANCY	EXPULSION	REMOVAL FOR BLEEDING/PAIN
All First Fittings	LOW 1.2 ± 0.6	MODERATE 8.8 ± 1.5	HIGH 18.3 ± 2.2
All Parous	LOW 1.2 ± 0.6	MODERATE 8.9 ± 1.6	HIGH 18.4 ± 2.2
Parity 1 & 2	LOW 0.8 ± 0.5	MODERATE 9.7 ± 1.9	HIGH 18.0 ± 2.6
Age — Under 30	LOW 1.4 ± 0.8	HIGH 10.5 ± 2.1	HIGH 17.4 ± 2.7
Age — 30 & Over	LOW 0.9 ± 0.8	MODERATE 5.6 ± 2.1	HIGH 19.9 ± 3.9
Under 30 Parity 1 & 2	LOW 1.1 ± 0.8	HIGH 11.9 ± 2.5	HIGH 18.7 ± 3.1

...sed on one year of use. Figures represent net event rates (with S.E.) per 100 users with at least 100 women remaining in ...e study during the twelfth month.

DALKON SHIELD

This device is made of polyvinyl acetate and contains barium sulphate (12 per cent), copper dust (0.45 − 0.55 per cent) and copper sulphate (0.9 − 1.1 per cent). Its design incorporates a series of lateral fins surrounding a central membrane. The fins are intended to promote retention of the device in the uterus and the central membrane increase the area of surface interaction between the device and the endometrium.

A.H. Robins Company Limited stopped marketing the Dalkon Shield in 1974 following reports from the United States of America of septic abortions, some of them fatal, among women who became pregnant while wearing this device. It has been suggested that infection was introduced into the uterus by means of the polyfilament tail attached to the IUD. All other currently available devices have monofilament tails. The Dalkon Shield is no longer generally available but a large number of women are still wearing this device in the United Kingdom at the present time. If a patient becomes pregnant and is believed to be wearing a Dalkon Shield, the device may reasonably be removed if the strings are visible and removal is easy even though the risk of spontaneous abortion appears to be increased as a result of the removal procedure.

COPPER OMEGA

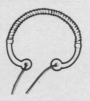

The development of the Copper Omega device commenced in 1969. The device consists of two smooth rounded heads connected to each other by a semicircular cross-member. The device is made of polypropylene and copper wire is wound around the cross-member which is serrated at even intervals to hold the wire in place.

There are four sizes of the Copper Omega. A trial certificate under the Medicines Act has been given for the use of this device but it has not, to date, been marketed on a large scale. Preliminary trial results have shown the device to possess low pregnancy and expulsion rates but higher than average removal rates.

MULTILOAD

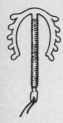

The Multiload is a polyethylene device 3.6 cm long with 27 cm of 0.3 mm diameter copper wire wound around its vertical stem. One model has 250 mm² of copper surface and a more recent version of the device has 375 mm² of copper surface. The device combines certain characteristics of the Dalkon Shield (spurs on the flexible arms) and of the Gyne T (vertical stem with copper wire wound around). The design of the Multiload attempts to combine ease of insertion, resistance to expulsion and a low pregnancy rate. Preliminary trials outside the United Kingdom indicate that this device has low pregnancy, expulsion, bleeding and pain removal rates.

PROGESTASERT

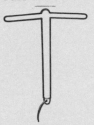

This recently introduced IUD is designed to deliver progesterone in the uterus at a rate of 65 µg/day. The device is a 'T' shaped unit with a reservoir of 38 mg progesterone in the vertical stem. The progesterone is dispersed in silicone oil and barium sulphate is added to render the dvice radio-opaque.

Information obtained in trials indicates that this device has similar pregnancy rates to other more conventional IUDs, though expulsion rates may be lower. The volume of blood loss appears to be reduced but the frequency of bleeding may be increased. This device requires replacement after each year of use but research continues with a view to devising a progesterone reservoir which will enable an extended duration of action.

Trials are in progress in the United Kingdom at the present time.

APPENDIX

THE SETTING UP OF AN IUD SERVICE

1. Equipment required.
2. Sterilisation of instruments and IUDs.
3. Follow-up administrative arrangements.
4. Loss to follow-up.
5. Recording system.
6. Assessment of IUD service.
7. Information to family doctor.
8. Training for provision of an IUD service in England and Wales.
9. Procedures for obtaining IUDs in England and Wales.
10. Payment for IUD service in England and Wales.

1. Equipment Required

The fitting doctor should possess:

Examination couch, preferably with lithotomy poles.
Sterile antiseptic solution.
Bivalve speculum.
Malleable uterine sound.
Long narrow (sponge) forceps.
Scissors (curved or straight).
Two single-toothed tenacula or a vulsellum.
Sterile cotton wool swabs.
Sterile disposable gloves.
Cervical dilators (Hegar).
Gräfenberg hook for removing device in the absence of a tail.
Bacteriological swabs and transport medium.
Spatula, slide and fixative (for Papanicolaou smear).
Facilities for the patient to lie down for 1 to 2 hours under observation should also be available in case of syncope, pain or bleeding at the time of IUD fitting or removal.

2. Sterilisation of Equipment

A sterile technique must be maintained throughout the fitting procedure. Most IUDs in general use come in a sterilised pack which minimises the risk of contamination. If the device, inserter (including the inner plunger and the outer sleeve) and other equipment used are not in a sterile condition they must be sterilised before fitting. Where there is no regular supply of sterile equipment, a steriliser will be needed for instruments. Do not boil or autoclave IUDs but use one of the known cold sterilisers such as benzalkonium chloride or aqueous iodine. Wash carefully in 0.1 per cent benzalkonium chloride and soak in the same for twenty-four hours or soak in 1.0 per cent benzalkonium chloride for six hours and then rinse in 0.1 per cent before use. Another method is to soak in diluted tincture of iodine or an iodine-iodide mixture with 0.04 per cent elemental iodine for five minutes and then rinse in sterile water. Plastic inserters lose their elasticity if boiled for prolonged periods of time.

3.   Follow-Up Schedule

Where no difficulties are encountered at IUD fitting, the patient should return to the clinic for a first follow-up visit within three months. The first three months of IUD use are known to be particularly important in relation to possible expulsion of the device and complaints relating to symptoms associated with heavy bleeding. A second follow-up visit should normally take place twelve months after fitting with annual visits thereafter. The IUD user should also be advised to return if she has any worries or symptoms associated with IUD use. It is important to ensure that the visits have a consistent pattern when preparing a follow-up schedule so that patients who are overdue for a scheduled visit can be easily identified. Strenuous efforts should be made to contact women who fail to keep their follow-up appointments.

4.   Loss to Follow-Up

This occurs when the patient fails to attend for a scheduled follow-up visit. Many doctors consider the follow-up of IUD patients to be the most difficult (and costly) part of an IUD service. Note should especially be made of patients wearing IUDs which require routine removal after stated time intervals (e.g. the copper-carrying or hormone-releasing IUDs). If these patients do not return for a follow-up visit, the risk of pregnancy may become considerable. Unlike other methods of contra-ception, the use of an IUD is not necessarily discontinued if the patient does not attend for follow-up.

5.   Recording System

The minimum record system can consist of a book in which the name of each IUD acceptor is entered together with her age, parity, date of IUD fitting, type of IUD fitted and brief details concerning subsequent follow-up visits. It is also advisable to note the date and reason for IUD discontinuation when this occurs. At a more sophisticated level an individual record card may be kept for each IUD acceptor. Information recorded on the card may include:

1.   Relevant details from the patient's medical and obstetric history;

2. Results of the pelvic examination and Papanicolaou smear when the device is fitted;
3. IUD fitting details (i.e. type of device, date of fitting, etc.);
4. Reports on each subsequent follow-up visit;
5. Date next follow-up visit is due; *or*
6. Date and reason for discontinuing use of the device.

It is useful to keep an additional index of names which are filed according to the month in which the woman is next due to attend for a follow-up visit. If she returns for the scheduled check visit her card is then replaced in the file in the month when her *next* follow-up visit is due. The cards remaining after the month concerned has passed will provide the names of those women who have not returned for a check visit and who are therefore technically lost to follow-up. Attempts should be made to contact these 'lost' patients by post, telephone or personal visit depending upon the resources and staff available for this purpose.

6. How to Assess the IUD Service

In the assessment of an IUD service it is important to obtain four sets of information:

1. Details of the patient.
2. Details of the IUD fitted.
3. Reasons for discontinuation of the method.
4. Months of IUD use.

1. Details of the Patient

The basic information required is the age and parity of the patient but additional facts can be recorded depending on the degree of refinement required. Other variables may include:

(i) occupational status of patient;
(ii) interval since last pregnancy or termination;
(iii) description of when in menstrual cycle the IUD was fitted;
(iv) whether a pregnancy is desired some time in the future;
(v) any difficulty in IUD fitting.

This list could be as extensive or as detailed as desired but care should be taken not to collect information which, owing to the small numbers involved, cannot by analysed accurately.

2. Details of the IUD

The IUD model and size should be recorded very carefully. A mistake is often made by doctors in a hurry and this may create problems later. New devices are introduced which bear a close resemblance to existing IUD models and care should be taken in distinguishing between them. Examples are the 'plain', 'wing' and 'film' Antigon, the three sizes of Saf-T-Coil and the four sizes of Lippes Loop.

3. **Reasons for IUD Discontinuation**

There are nine reasons or 'events' usually described for IUD discontinuation. These are:

(i)   unplanned pregnancy
(ii)   expulsion (partial or total)
(iii) removal
    a) following complaints of bleeding and/or pain;
    b) other 'medical' complaints by patient;
    c) patient wishes to have a pregnancy;
    d) other 'personal' reasons of the patient;
    e) doctor's choice (e.g. routine change or where doctor believes it advisable to remove IUD but no complaint has been made by the patient);
(iv)   patient released from follow-up
(v)   patient lost to follow-up.

The definitions of some of these events are given in more detail at the beginning of Section II of this manual.

It should be remembered that at any given time, a large proportion of IUD patients will continue to wear the IUD without one of the above 'events' taking place. Information relating to this satisfactory use of the IUD is equally important in the assessment of the IUD service.

4. **Months of IUD Use**

For each patient, the number of months, to the nearest month, between IUD fitting and a reported 'event' or between IUD fitting and the cut-off date selected for analysis, whichever occurs sooner, should be calculated. These 'months of use' are an important statistic in the calculation of IUD effectiveness rates.

Analysis of Data

There are several ways of measuring the efficiency of a contraceptive method. The simplest technique is to calculate the proportion of women experiencing a defined event such as an unplanned pregnancy among the total number of users of the method. This technique has a serious flaw in that it does not take into account the varying lengths of time the method has been in use. The event rate associated with IUDs which have been worn for a considerable length of time will be overstated in comparison to the event rate for devices worn only for a short period.

In 1932, Pearl introduced a method of measuring effectiveness which takes into account the length of time the patient has been exposed to the risk of a defined event. Known as the Pearl Index, the calculation is expressed in terms of a rate per 100 women years of exposure (abbreviated as HWY). The method of calculation is as follows:

$$\text{Rate per HWY} = \frac{\text{Total number of defined events} \times 1200}{\text{Total months of exposure to event risk}}$$

The denominator includes the total months of IUD use for all patients using the IUD model being assessed. Using the Pearl Index it is possible to compare the relative efficiency of two or more methods (or IUD models) even though the women are using each method for differing lengths of time.

One disadvantage of the Pearl Index is that it assumes that the monthly probability of an event remains constant over a period of time. Long-term studies of IUD use have demonstrated that this assumption is incorrect.

The more sophisticated life-table approach, which is similar to the technique used by life insurance companies in assessing risks, permits the calculation of a rate concerning a specific risk (e.g. pregnancy) over a defined period of time taking into account the presence of other competing risks (e.g. removal and expulsion) during the same period of time. It also assesses the changing probability of risk for defined events over a period of time. The calculations are expressed in terms of a rate per 100 women after n months or years of observation. Application of the life-table approach involves fairly complicated statistical procedures and computer facilities may be required. Advice should be sought before embarking on this type of analysis.

The Pearl Index may be a cruder indicator than life-table rates but providing the number of cases is reasonably large, and the period of time that the IUD is used averages out at more than a year for each patient, the Pearl Index obtained permits useful comparisons between contraceptive methods or IUD models.

7. Information to Family Doctor

If the IUD patient is not the doctor's own patient, the family doctor must be informed that the patient is wearing an IUD, provided the patient will give her permission for this to be done. The IUD model and size should also be specified. The treatment of side effects reported to the family doctor and the management of a possible pregnancy when wearing the IUD may depend on the type of IUD being worn.

If the patient will not allow her family doctor to be informed, then it is incumbent on the doctor fitting the IUD to provide a 24-hour procedure to deal with any emergency complication that may arise.

8. **Training for Provision of an IUD Service**

It is essential that practical training in the fitting of IUDs should be undertaken by those contemplating the fitting of IUDs. Area Health Authorities are responsible for organising training courses on contraceptive services. The syllabus for these courses is approved by the Joint Committee on Contraception of the Royal College of General Practitioners, the Royal College of Obstetricians, Gynaecologists, the Family Planning Association and the National Association of Family Planning Doctors. These courses usually involce two days of theoretical instruction on contraceptive techniques — including the IUD — and a number of practical sessions (about eight) in a recognised training clinic. Supervised insertion of IUDs is required during the practical training sessions. Upon satisfactory completion of the course the trainee is granted a certificate by the Joint Committee on Contraception. Information about training courses may be obtained from the Area Medical Officer of the Area Health Authority.

9. **Procedures for Obtaining IUDs in England and Wales**

Intrauterine devices included on the National Health Service drug tariff are available to women by prescription on Form FP10. At the present time the Lippes Loop, the Saf-T-Coil and the Gravigard device (Copper 7) are the only IUDs listed on the drug tariff. A prescription charge is not levied for these devices. Clinic and hospital services are supplied with devices by the Area Health Authority and may include devices not listed on the National Health Service drug tariff. Other devices can be purchased directly from the distributors concerned but it may also be useful to seek information from the Area Medical Officer of the Area Health Authority.

10. **Payment for the IUD Service in England and Wales**

Within the National Health Service, a doctor is required to apply to the local Family Practitioner Committee for his name to be included on the list of those providing a contraceptive service if he wishes to provide such a service. In making this application the doctor should indicate whether or not he wishes to restrict contraceptive services to his own patients and whether or not he wishes to fit intrauterine devices. There are separate forms for claiming the ordinary fee for contraceptive services (FP 1001) and for claiming the intrauterine device fee (FP 1002). Both fees are fixed as annual rates payable for services given over a twelve-month period but the rates are different.

The ordinary contraceptive fee covers payment for advice on the choice of method, services required in the provision of female methods (excluding the IUD) and any necessary aftercare associated with these methods. An intrauterine device fee is payable for services provided in the twelve months commencing from the date an IUD is fitted. The IUD fee is not supplementary to the ordinary contraceptive fee and the IUD fee is only payable if the doctor himself, his partner or assistant fits the device and provides the necessary aftercare, including refitting if necessary, during the twelve months following the first IUD fitting. Twelve months after the first IUD fitting the ordinary fee becomes payable for any subsequent period during which the IUD fitted in the first year continues to be worn by the patient. If the patient is refitted with another IUD after this twelve month period, the process starts again as if she were a new patient.

Doctors are precluded from issuing National Health Service prescriptions for private patients for contraceptive substances or appliances including intrauterine devices.

The Family Practitioner Notice and Statement of Fees and Allowances issued by the Department of Health and Social Security should be consulted for additional information about payment for contraceptive services. Any enquiries concerning this document should be addressed to the Family Practitioner Committee in the Area Health Authority. The forms which enable patients to apply for contraceptive services and doctors to claim a fee are supplied by this Committee.

USEFUL REFERENCES

Davis, H.J. (1971), *Intrauterine Devices for Contraception: The IUD*. Williams and Wilkins, Baltimore.

Elder, M.G., Hawkins, D.F. (1977), *Human Fertility Control: Theory and Practice*. Butterworths, London.

Hefnawi, F., Segal, S.J. (1975), *Analysis of Intrauterine Contraception* North-Holland/American Elsevier, New York.

Kleinman, R.L. (1977), *Intrauterine Contraception*. IPPF, London.

Oldershaw, K.L. (1975), *Contraception, Abortion and Sterilization in General Practice*. Henry Kimpton, London.

Population Reports, Series B, *Intrauterine Devices*. Department of Medical and Public Affairs, The George Washington University Medical Center, Washington, D.C.

Ramaswamy, S., Smith, A. (1976), *Practical Contraception*. Pitman Medical, Tunbridge Wells, Kent.

Tatum, H.J. (1977), Clinical Aspects of Intrauterine Contraception: Circumspection 1976, *Fertility and Sterility*. Vol. 28, no. 1.

Tietze, C., Lewit, S. (1973), Recommended Procedures for the Statistical Evaluation of Intrauterine Contraception, *Studies in Family Planning*. Vol. 4, no. 2; or *Clinical Obstetrics and Gynecology*. (1974), vol. 17, no. 1.

Wheeler, R.G., Duncan, G.W., Speidel, J.J. (1974), *Intrauterine Device* Academic Press, New York, London.

Wishik, S., Hulka, J.F. (1970), *Casebook for the Intrauterine Contraceptive Device*. International Institute for the Study of Human Reproduction, Columbia University.

Wood, C. (1971), *Intrauterine Devices*. Butterworths, London.

USEFUL ADDRESSES

Lippes Loop
Gyne T (Copper T)

Ortho Pharmaceutical Ltd
P.O. Box 79
Saunderton
High Wycombe
Bucks. HP14 4HJ.

Saf-T-Coil

LR Industries Ltd
North Circular Road
London E4 8QA.

Gravigard (Copper 7)

G.D. Searle & Co Ltd
P.O. Box 53
Lane End Road
High Wycombe
Bucks. HP12 4HL.

Antigon

Svend Schroder
112 Bjerringbrovej
Rodovre
Denmark.

Copper Omega

EMM – IUD Ltd
22 South Parade
Southsea
Hants. PO5 2JF.

Progestasert

May & Baker Ltd
Dagenham
Essex.

Multiload

J. van Brunschot b.v.
Spinozastraat 47
Amsterdam C
Netherlands.

Information on
Dalkon Shield

A.H. Robins Co Ltd
1407 Cummings Drive
Richmond
Virginia, USA.